Your Fourth Choice

Your
Fourth
Choice

Killing Cancer Cells with
PAW PAW
That Little-Known Treatment
that Grows on Trees

—○—

John Clifton

Foley Square, New York

Publication date: April, 2015. ISBN: 978-0-9760846-9-3
Library of Congress Control Number: Pending

Additional copies and information:
Visit our web site at *www.YourFourthChoice.com* for further information, continuously updated resources on paw paw, and to order additional copies of this book. Also, you will find at the very end of this book a mail-in order form for purchasing more copies.

ATTENTION: UNIVERSITIES, COLLEGES, and PROFESSIONAL and CHARITABLE ORGANIZATIONS: Quantity discounts are available on bulk purchases of this book for educational and gift purposes, or as premiums in fundraising efforts. Inquiries should be addressed to:

Foley Square Books, 175 West 87th Street, Room 27E
New York, NY 10024   212-724-1578
info@FoleySquareBooks.com

Look deep into nature, and then you will
understand everything better.
—Albert Einstein

For Glenn, Harold, and Thelma

Contents

Preface

The idea for this book came out of frustration—and not a little anger. Up to about 150 years ago *all* medicine was natural, derived from natural material—plant, animal, and mineral. There was no "alternative" division as opposed to "standard" medicine. People today, though, seem to fall into one of three categories regarding cancer: (1) those who trust in standard medicine only—rejecting all alternative or natural treatment, (2) those who mistrust standard medicine and completely endorse natural remedies, and (3) those who are somewhere in the middle, having no hard and fast opinions about either side.

If I had to categorize myself, I suppose I would fall into the third group—although I do have some strong opinions.

Standard treatments at least have the validation of extensive testing, clinical trials, survival data, etc., and a more solid sense of "you know what to expect."

Alternative medicines rely more upon anecdotal evidence—this case and that case, this story and that story of patients and their experiences with particular natural remedies. Not that there haven't been trials and studies regarding natural medicines—there have, but certainly the Alternative side can't compete with the millions of dollars that the Standard side pours into research, product development, not to mention *promotion* of their products.

When I, through personal experience and research, became aware of the startling effectiveness of a natural remedy called "paw paw" I felt both the thrill of discovery and the frustration of realizing that most people knew little or nothing about it.

"Big Pharma"—the gigantic pharmaceutical industry— has spent fortunes on convincing us that their products are effective, safe, tested, standard, unassailable, wonderful, amazing—*and*—covered by insurance!

And of course, these big drugs are legally protected, both under patent law and through legal disclaimers regarding side effects, etc. Sometimes their commercials devote more time to warnings about a drug than its benefits. "If death occurs, stop taking *Amazitol* and call your doctor."

No wonder that Nature is on the losing side. And no wonder that many people mistrust natural products—they simply haven't been bombarded with expensive commercial messages about them.

To be clear, I'm talking about natural *medicines*—not vitamins and dietary supplements. These indeed receive their share of attention in the marketplace of health products. Perhaps too much attention—to the extent that many well-intentioned people are indiscriminately popping all sorts of vitamin and mineral pills that they don't always need. Much of their money (and those pills) are going down the drain, so to speak.

Then there is the quackery factor. We've all heard stories about totally bogus—even harmful—products being touted as "cures" for you-name-it, and particularly cancer. So people are doubly cautious, and rightly so.

When I became aware of the benefits of paw paw, I wanted to share what I knew to—well—to the world! And the result is this modest handbook on a little-known cancer treatment that is, in my opinion, abundantly worth knowing about.

What you will find here is a simple guide to paw paw—a natural cancer remedy with a solid background of research, and supported by much evidence.

I will explain just what paw paw is, where it comes from and how it could benefit anyone with cancer of most any type. I will tell, in simple understandable terms, how it works in the body. I'll give you a brief history of its development, how it's been tested, researched, etc. I will keep it simple, non-technical, and straightforward.

I'll tell you where to get paw paw, how much (little!) it is likely to cost, how to use it, and how much to take. I'll try to convey how fighting cancer is more than passively putting oneself in the hands of the medical profession—and requires personal initiative.

It is my hope that this book will introduce many cancer victims (and hopefully their doctors) to an alternative that could extend their lives and possibly even save their lives.

—o—

I'll begin with a personal account. . . .

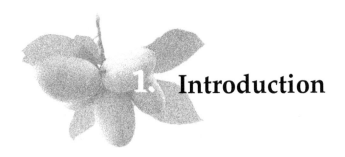

1. Introduction

Josée's story

Chances are you've never heard of paw paw. I know I hadn't, and my wife Josée hadn't—not until she got cancer, in the fall of 2012. Josée was diagnosed with endometrial cancer, which is cancer of the walls of the uterus.

Her gynecologist scheduled her for a hysterectomy, but in the screening process for the operation some irregularities showed up on her chest x-ray. She was then referred to a pulmonologist who did further testing and imaging. He found some masses in her right lung and also some suspicious nodules in her left lung.

So the next stop was an oncologist. After more testing, more scans, and several biopsies the verdict came in: Stage Four non-small cell lung cancer. Just the kind of diagnosis you never want to hear. The survival rate of Stage Four lung cancer is next to zero. And the bad news just happened to come on the day of Christmas Eve. Some present!

The lung cancer was totally unrelated to the uterine cancer—they were two separate, simultaneous cancers. The main mass was in her right lung, and measured 3.5 centimeters in diameter. There were metastases in some lymph nodules, and further malignancy throughout her left lung.

Josée was immediately put on standard chemotherapy. It was presented to us as "palliative" treatment—meaning there was no expectation of a cure, but the cancer could be brought "under control" and she would enjoy a better "quality of life." And she might live somewhat longer than she could expect to *without* the chemo.

So the treatments were started, and we would just have to hope for the best. Josée's primary care doctor advised to try to accept the situation and "enjoy life" and the days that were left.

But I just couldn't accept sitting back and waiting for some kind of inevitable doomsday. And battling cancer was nothing new to us. Our dog Sparky[1] had contracted canine lymphoma (deadly in dogs) when he was six years old back in 2001, and we had gotten him through that. What we learned was that miracles *can* happen—but you have to help them along; you have to open doors so that the miracles can pass through.[2] Sparky lived, cancer-free, to the ripe old age of fourteen and a half—we weren't going to take this Stage-Four-lung-cancer-thing lying down!

The search for alternative answers

Since standard medicine was not offering a cure, I decided to investigate everything I could *outside of* traditional by-the-book treatment. And, boy, was there a lot of it! Nutritional supplements, anti-oxidants, special formulas of all kinds, cancer diets, etc., etc., etc.

Here's a sampling of what's out there:

Alpha Lipoic Acid	Cannabis
Artemisinin	CoQ10
BLA Elixir	Curcumin

Dichloroacetate (DCA)	Omega-3 fatty acids
Enzymes	Omega-6 Oils
Fish Oil	OxyDHQ
Garlic	Protocel
Ginger	Ronuv
Green tea	Selenium
L-glutamine	Sodium Bicarbonate (to reduce bodily acidity)
Life Force Elixir (energized water)	Super PEO
Liquid Zeolite (removes toxic metals)	Vitamin D

Well, you get the idea. The list could go on endlessly. I looked up all these things and more, collecting the information in a three-ring binder—thinking, weighing, considering, evaluating—desperately looking for the magic bullet that might be the answer to beating Josée's cancers. Artemisinin looked especially good—there were many amazing cases involving that ancient Chinese herb. (I recommend that you look that one up!) I had heard about curcumin, the kitchen spice that kills cancer cells. And of course there's the matter of diet—what do you eat to fight cancer and what do you avoid?

Cancer cells, I learned, thrive on carbohydrates and sugar. Starve them! Eat vegetables and lean meats and fish. Oh great, I thought—this is going to really upset our lives. What's more ingrained than your eating habits? Give up bread? The very thought was daunting. Josée and I are seniors, and pretty set in our ways. We just couldn't imagine ourselves tolerating the radical changes this literature was insisting we make.

The first oncologist we had consulted maintained that there's no proof that *any* of this stuff worked. No blind studies, no serious research. Just go with chemotherapy; nothing but standard treatments could be trusted. (Surgery, of course was out with this sort of metastasized cancer, as was radiation, due to the widespread areas of the tumors.)

So, that's the catch. Standard medicine promises no cure, but it's the only thing that has been studied, and therefore all you should go for. Hmm.

Not all oncologists agree with this, in cases like Josée's. In fact we found that our next oncologist, who was to be our main man, was open to whatever "extra-curricular" treatments we might come up with.

So I persisted on my search for that one standout alternative treatment that (a) looked promising and (b) had at least *some* validation through tests and anecdotal accounts.

Then one day I just happened to notice a meme someone had posted on Facebook. It was about "graviola," a tropical fruit that was purported to shrink tumors. Someone had commented below the meme that "paw paw" worked even better than graviola.

"Paw paw?" What was that? Another name for papaya? I looked it up. No, paw paw is not papaya. I was intrigued, and proceeded to investigate the matter. Perhaps it would be worth a try. So, what is paw paw anyway? I'll tell you in the next chapter what I found out.

The treatments begin

Meanwhile, Josée began her first chemotherapy sequence. She would have infusions every three weeks, starting in February of 2013. Her treatments would consist basically of two agents, Carboplatin[3] and Paclitaxel[4]—more or less standard for lung cancer patients. She would also be given Neupogen,[5] a drug to boost the white blood cells destroyed by the chemotherapy.

Along the way she began taking paw paw. We told her oncologist about this and he had no objection. This doctor was very open-minded about her interest in alternative treatments, although, as most oncologists, he knew very little about them. Medical schools teach only three treatments for cancer: chemotherapy, radiation, and surgery. Those are the Standard Medicine Big Three, and oncologists have been taught little else.

The paw paw started some time in March. By May, Josée had had four chemotherapy sessions and it was time for a CT scan ("CAT scan") of her torso, from her neck down to her upper legs. This would include her uterus as well as the lungs. (The uterine cancer was not treated separately—it just went along for the ride, so to speak, and was expected to react to the chemo along with the lungs.) Since lung cancer tends to spread to the brain, Josée also had a brain MRI.

We were both holding our breath to see the results of these scans. The oncologist had warned us—and our reading on the topic confirmed—that lung cancer was tough to control. It tends to spread to other parts of the body. Chemotherapy was trying to put a lid on it, while the cancer was pushing to expand.

Well, it was an amazing session with the doctor. He told us that the main mass in her right lung had greatly reduced in size, and that the metastases in her left lung weren't there anymore. "We don't see them," he said. He was amazed, and we were delighted. It was a very happy day!

A few weeks later we had another appointment with the oncologist. He had been consulting with colleagues, and brought up the possibility of surgery, since there was basically only one mass remaining—in the right lung— along with a few nearby lymph nodes. We consulted with a surgeon. But he was hesitant to operate on a 78-year-old patient if there was another option. The other option was radiation.

So we met with a radiologist, and began targeted radiation treatments simultaneously with another round of chemo—this time "Alimta."[6]

But midway through the series, Josée became so toxic that the chemo and radiation had to be stopped. She could barely swallow, and suffered pains and extreme nausea. Her oncologist called an end to it all. But she continued to take the paw paw, and suffered no ill effects from that. Six weeks went by, with no treatment, only paw paw. She then had a scheduled PET scan.[7]

No cancer was seen. She had a biopsy done on the endometrial cancer as well. Negative.

Of course, lung cancer has a way of eventually coming back. As I write this, it's late in the year 2014, and so far it hasn't shown up.

This was such an amazing result! We are convinced that the paw paw had a lot to do with it. It's claimed that paw paw kills cancer cells that chemotherapy leaves behind. Is this true? Was Josée's case consistent with others who had taken paw paw? How did this stuff work? What was going on?

What trials had been conducted? What had other users of paw paw experienced?

Those questions will be what this book is about.

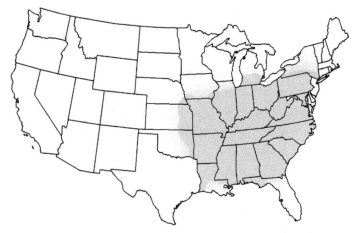

Where Paw Paw Grows in the United States

(Shaded area)

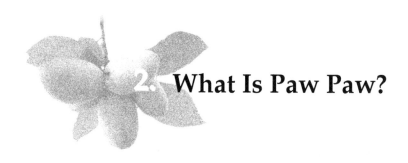

2. What Is Paw Paw?

Paw Paw is the name of a tree. There are several species, but the one we'll concern ourselves with here bears the Latin name *Asimina triloba.*[8] Paw paw trees bear an edible fruit. I've personally never tasted paw paw, but they say it tastes something like banana, and people who are fortunate to have a paw paw tree in their backyard really like the tasty fruit. The trees typically aren't very big. The fruits are light greenish-yellow and are about the size of mangos and similar in overall shape.

There are natural substances found in the paw paw tree that are the key to its anti-cancer properties. They are called *acetogenins.* Acetogenins are the key medicinal operatives in paw paw. In the next chapter, we'll examine acetogenins more closely.

Where does paw paw grow?

The trees are found in North America, especially in the eastern United States. So, you see, they are not tropical—although they do have some tropical relatives. Ironically, my wife Josée Clerens had written a book about the Louisiana Purchase[9] several years ago, and in describing the western wilderness she listed "paw paw" among the indigenous trees. Little did she know how important that tree would become in her life!

The main reason people aren't familiar with the fruit is that it's not available in grocery stores. And the reason for *that* is that paw paw doesn't travel well, and tends to spoil after it's picked. So if you want to taste paw paw you'll most likely have to find or grow a paw paw tree! Not that the fruit is the important part of the tree, medicinally speaking. Actually, it's the *twigs* that bear the most plentiful amounts of the powerful acetogenins—but more about that later.

Is paw paw the same as graviola?

Graviola (A*nnona muricata)* is a tropical tree—a relative of paw paw—and with similar medicinal qualities. But graviola has nowhere *near* the strength and power of paw paw. To be sure, graviola does have anticancer properties, and many cancer patients have benefited from it.[10] Tests were done, however, to compare graviola with paw paw— and paw paw came out the hands-down winner.[11]

Is paw paw a "Miracle Cure?"

I'm always leery about any product that claims to be a "miracle." When I see an ad for a product something along the lines of "Dr. Quackenbush's Miracle Elixir" I'm immediately repelled. There is no magic bullet, no sure cure for cancer. Nothing works in all cases, nor works to the same degree in all patients.

But treating cancer shouldn't be a crap shoot either. Some things have proven to work more often, and on more people, than others. Standard medicine is based on clinical trials as well as statistics and track records of each treatment. There are data to show what percentages of which people (with certain ages, backgrounds, gender, medical history, etc.) respond to certain treatments.

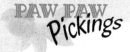

What's in a Name?

The name "paw paw" sounds like it might be a Native American word, but more likely it came from "papaya," a tropical fruit tree and a distant relative of the North American paw paw tree.

Major clinical trials are needed in order to attain government approval for every drug and treatment used. This research costs *millions* of dollars for each drug/treatment studied. New drugs, then, require major investments to be made by the pharmaceutical companies. And these companies are not going to invest unless they will be able to maintain patents over the drugs and treatments.

Natural remedies cannot in themselves be patented. You can't patent something that literally "grows on trees." You might patent a *process* on how it's manufactured, extracted, etc., but you can't patent the stuff itself. One might say that Nature holds the patent! What the drug companies often *can* do is synthesize the natural element so that it can be reproduced chemically. *This* can be patented. For example, the chemotherapy agent *Paclitaxel* was derived and synthesized from natural compounds found in the bark of the Pacific yew tree.

The acetogenins in Paw paw, however, have not been found to be economically synthesizable. Hence, "Big Pharma" is not interested. Therefore there have been no million-dollar clinical studies done on paw paw. *But that is not to say that there haven't been any studies.* In fact, there have been several, and in addition, much anecdotal evidence showing the benefits of paw paw and its acetogenins. I'll show you some specific examples later on.

Which brings us to the answer to the question: Is paw paw a "miracle cure?" I would have to say no, not always—but the paw paw *tree* certainly is a miracle *tree*!

And, personally, paw paw has been a miracle for many people.

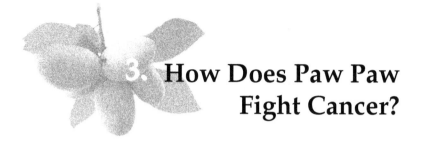

3. How Does Paw Paw Fight Cancer?

How do cells make energy?

All cells, both normal and cancerous, need energy to survive. We feed our bodies with food, and our bodies digest the food, transforming it into forms that cells can use—to live, grow, and multiply. One of the main substances produced by digestion is ... sugar! Yes, much of our food is changed into glucose—a sugar that cells thrive on. Cancer cells, in particular, love glucose—it's their favorite fuel.

Cells have a mechanism for selecting glucose and oxygen from our blood and transporting these into their interior.

But cells can't really use glucose and oxygen "as is." They have to change it into a form of energy they can use. They take the oxygen and glucose and process these into another substance. This substance is very, very important—and has a name to match: *adenosine triphosphate.* Hard to remember? Just call it by its nickname, ATP.

In a nutshell, the process goes like this:

Elements in food are turned into blood

Blood carries glucose and oxygen to cells

Cells change glucose and oxygen into energy (ATP)

Cells use energy to sustain themselves, grow, and multiply

Now, *cancer* cells need much more energy than normal cells. They tend to grow faster and multiply faster than normal cells. If we could just deprive them of their ability to *produce* that energy we could arrest the progress of cancer. So, what's in cells that enables them to produce ATP (energy)? That would be (sorry to use another ten-dollar word) the *mitochondria.*

What are mitochondria and why are they important to cancer cells?

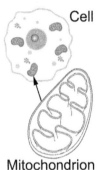
Cell

Mitochondrion

Within every cell there are thousands (*hundreds* of thousands!) of mitochondria—little sausage-shaped structures—one of whose jobs it is to produce ATP from the glucose and oxygen. Mitochondria are found in all cells—both cancerous and normal. The thing is, cancerous cells need a lot more energy than normal ones. As noted, they grow faster and reproduce faster. Their mitochondria are doing extra heavy duty!

By now you may be wondering what all this has to do with paw paw. Well, there are particular operatives in paw paw that actually attack the mitochondria. . . .

Just what are "acetogenins?"

The paw paw tree—the fruit, the leaves, the branches—produces compounds called *acetogenins*, as I mentioned earlier. It has been discovered that these acetogenins actually *reduce* the ability of the mitochondria to produce energy.[12] Without mitochondria producing the energy they need, the cells weaken and *die.* The acetogenins in paw paw seek out the fastest-growing cells, and pretty much ignore the normal cells.[13]

Do any standard medicines attack mitochondria in cancer cells?"

Historically, in conventional medicine, it was thought that the mitochondria were not important in cancer cells' metabolic processes. Cancer cells, it was believed, while they still contained (dysfunctional) mitochondria, relied on a process called "glycolysis" as the major metabolic pathway. Mitochondria were just not important where tumorous cells were concerned. So you can see that a medicine which attacked the mitochondria would not have been considered effective in stopping the proliferation of tumor cells—glycolysis was doing the metabolizing (creating the energy), and that was that. It's no wonder that *not a single standard chemotherapy drug works on the principle of attacking mitochondria.*

Today it is accepted that mitochondrial metabolism is *essential* for cancer cell proliferation. And the mitochondria are functional in almost all cancer cells. There are a very few cells that might be relying solely upon glycolysis for their metabolic process. But *even these cells* depend upon the contribution made by the presence of mitochondria!

And here's the kicker—now that all this is known, they are thinking about developing medicines to attack the mitochondria! One recent article (2014) on the topic sums up with this sentence:

> Collectively, these insights have led to the possibility of targeting mitochondria for cancer therapy.[14]

Well, *duhh!* Paw paw has been known to do this very thing for over thirty years. Think for a moment what this says about the state of standard medicine today!

What are multiple drug resistant (MDR) cells and how does paw paw kill them?

When cancer is treated with traditional chemotherapy it is often the case that a few cells become resistant (immune) to the chemotherapy. These are called MDR (Multiple Drug Resistant) cells. Notice the word "multiple." Cells treated with one chemotherapy drug may become resistant to other drugs as well. There may be a very small number of these resistant cells remaining after a cycle of chemo. But remember that cancer cells divide and multiply. One or two cells can soon become a new malignant mass.

MDR cells actually develop mechanisms that simply expel the chemotherapy drugs. They actually pump the drug out of the cell. This accounts for the fact that so many cancer cases are never finally cured by chemotherapy. A patient may look cancer-free on a diagnostic scan,

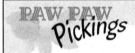

Please Don't Feed the Cancer Cells

Cells take in glucose from the blood and the mitochondria in the cells transform the glucose into energy (ATP). Cancer cells, according to studies, need 10-17 times as much ATP as normal cells in order to survive!

and then the cancer returns. This is due to those MDR cells that have survived the chemo treatment.

Paw paw works differently. Chemo is basically a poison, and the body can develop immunity to poisons. (Think about people who take a tiny quantity of snake venom, then gradually increase the quantity, the result being that they eventually become immune to snake bites.) Paw paw is not a strong poison—the body does not become immune to it. Paw paw can actually *kill* MDR cells. Because it deprives cells of energy, paw paw weakens the MDR cells, depriving them of the energy needed to pump the chemo out! This is one reason why paw paw can be so effective when used in conjunction with standard chemotherapy. It can clean up the cells that chemo leaves behind.

Just think about that for a moment, and you can see the amazing benefit that paw paw can provide!

Is paw paw anti-angiogenic?

The simple answer to this question is "yes."

One of the modes used in treating cancer involves killing or inhibiting the growth of the blood vessels that transport energy from the bloodstream into the cancer cells. The process of growing blood vessels is called "angiogenesis." The process of inhibiting the growth of blood vessels is called *anti*-angiogenesis.

Just as cancer cells need energy (ATP) to thrive, so do the nearby blood vessels that supply them. Remember that cancer cells need *more* energy than normal cells. For this reason, cancer cells have to develop new blood vessels in order to boost the supply. This growth also needs ATP—just like new cancer cells do. So this is another way that blood vessels prevents the growth of cancer.[15]

—o—

By now you may be wondering how treating cancer with paw paw came about, and how we discovered all the surprising qualities and capabilities of this humble American tree. That's next. . . .

4. How Did Paw Paw Develop as a Cancer Treatment?

Who is behind the research?

To know the background and developmental history of paw paw is to know the work of paw paw's most prominent researcher and advocate, Jerry McLaughlin, Professor Emeritus of Pharmacognosy[16] at Purdue University. Dr. McLaughlin (presently retired) has devoted three decades of his life to the study of the paw paw tree and its medical uses.

Dr. McLaughlin's early interest was in graviola—that aforementioned tropical tree which, like paw paw, contains acetogenins. McLaughlin and his research team,[17] interested in graviola's cytotoxic (anti-cancer) properties, were able to isolate more than twenty-eight compounds found in graviola.

The study of graviola led naturally to paw paw, another tree in the family of plants known as *Annonaceae*. It was found that paw paw held more powerful cytotoxic properties than graviola. There are more than one species of paw paw, but it was found that one particular species—*Asimina triloba* provided the highest concentrations of those very special cancer-fighting acetogenins. The most obvious part of the tree to initially test was the fruit, which is edible and quite pleasant tasting. But further analysis led to the discovery that the *twigs* held the highest potency, containing more acetogenins than other parts of the tree. Furthermore, it was discovered that the acetogenin levels peaked in a certain month! That month was May, and consequently it is during that month that the twigs are harvested.

The studies are very detailed and exhaustive. It was even discovered that trees in certain groves of paw paw were more powerful than trees in other groves. The study of paw paw, as you can see, has been thorough, detailed, extremely scientific, and reliable. The more you look into it, the more you discover—and the more you become aware of the wealth of information and data that has been produced (more on the studies in the next chapter).

Why isn't paw paw a "standard" protocol?

You may now be asking; if there has been so much research and evidence that paw paw is effective and safe, why has it not been adopted as a standard treatment?

Good question.

The answer involves understanding the process of getting new treatments approved for use by the federal government. Every new drug coming down the pike, before being approved as an effective treatment by the Federal Drug Administration (FDA) must go through rigorous testing—through intensive (and expensive!) clinical trials. These trials, as noted earlier, cost millions. (Note the difference between a trial and a study. Paw paw has been studied extensively, but still awaits a clinical trial on humans.)

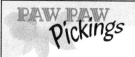

Celebrating Paw Paw

An annual event in Albany, Ohio, the *Ohio Paw Paw Festival* is a fun-filled and educational community event celebrating "one of America's largest native tree fruits," the Paw Paw. This three-day event highlights the rich history and future possibilities of the paw paw through delectable foods, quality entertainment, unique arts, crafts, and local businesses throughout southeastern Ohio and beyond.

http://ohiopawpawfest.com/about.html

So, if a pharmaceutical company is going to invest millions, it has to have the expectation that the drug will make those millions back—to pay for the trials and make a profit beyond that. And the only way to make sure that others don't profit from the investment made in developing and testing the drug is to *get a patent on it.*

It is often the case that a new drug starts from a natural substance—I mentioned before that the chemotherapy drug *Paclitaxel* was developed from a substance found in the bark of a yew tree. You can't patent a known natural substance, but what you *can* do is synthesize it chemically. The synthesized product, then, can be patented—and you don't have to bother anymore with the natural source from which it was synthesized. You make it in a laboratory.

But not all natural substances lend themselves to this kind of chemical replication. The acetogenins in paw paw are among those substances. Therefore no one is going to invest the fortunes necessary for massive clinical trials. Without

FDA approval, paw paw purveyors can't even use the word "cancer" in describing their product!

Personally, it's one of my pet peeves (outrages!) that the process of approving new drugs is exclusively profit-oriented. Nothing wrong with the profit motive—however there are many effective natural remedies that deserve government approval, but since they cannot be patented they never get trials, and hence never get approved. Why isn't there any government money allocated to testing promising non-patentable drugs?

Further, there is much distrust among many cancer victims, I have found, in anything classified as "alternative." I have personally recommended paw paw (and other natural products) to cancer patients of my acquaintance and, in spite of the example of my wife's success, they would not even consider any treatment not bearing the stamp of traditional medicine—even though that traditional medicine promises them not-so-great odds of beating their cancer!

In a rather recent study of cancer victims in Australia and the United States,[18] the *overall* cancer cure rate (defined as surviving past five years after diagnosis) was seen to be about 68%. In the same study, the cure rate for *chemotherapy* was determined to be 2.1%. In looking at all the data, one can't help but get the impression that alternative treatments do *far* better than traditional chemotherapy. Yet we are being led to believe that chemo is the tried and true way to go!

We are all simply obligated to explore alternative treatments if we would maximize survival. But this in turn obligates us to be selective, relying upon solid information, and avoiding hype.

Most all the information about paw paw that's readily available to the public is found on the Internet (and even there, it's not extensive). Online sources, of course, can be notoriously wrong, and much of the medical advice on websites is purely there to sell a product. Most people have built up a healthy suspicion of much medical information found online. The good, responsible information is co-mingled with the quackery. It is my hope that this book will help to remedy this predicament so far as paw paw and its use against cancer are concerned. Somehow, and perhaps mostly for good reason, the printed word is taken more seriously than something read on a computer screen.

The following section provides some more concrete data on the cancer-fighting properties of paw paw in actual use. Naturally, exhaustive clinical trials would help—but there's an abundance of positive evidence nonetheless.

—o—

Let's see some of that evidence. . . .

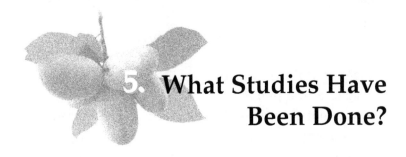

5. What Studies Have Been Done?

Paw Paw isn't some new drug that's just hit the scene. Its cancer-fighting properties have been studied for several decades. Many, many people have already benefited from it, and there is a wealth of documentation, tests, trials, studies and scientific articles—all centered upon this amazing natural substance. In fact, it could be said that among all "alternative" treatments paw paw is by far the most studied. It's beyond the scope of *Your Fourth Choice* to provide extensive amounts of scientific details. For those seeking more detailed medical/technical information, I refer you to the *References* section near the end of this book.

Early experiments

Way back in the Stone Age (circa 1976), Jerry L. McLaughlin, the aforementioned pharmacognosist at Purdue University, became interested in the paw paw, a tree he had known of since childhood. Dr. McLaughlin's special interest was in the medicinal qualities of plants, and he began to turn his attention to the paw paw tree. He was especially interested in toxicology—the study of poisons—and how it related to pharmacology—the study of drugs. He observed that "pharmacology is simply toxicology at a lower dose."[19]

McLaughlin decided to expose some brine shrimp to an extract of paw paw twigs. The brine shrimp dropped like flies. Compared to an equal amount of strychnine, paw paw did a far better job of killing the brine shrimp! McLaughlin and his team were able to isolate one of the acetogenins in paw paw that was the responsible party: *asimicin*. Turns out that this asimicin also proved "lethal to blowfly larvae, two-spotted spider mites, Mexican bean beetles, mosquito larvae, melon aphids, striped cucumber beetles and a nematode."[20]

The next natural step was to begin testing in laboratory animals. In one particular instance, certain acetogenins in paw paw were found to be more powerful in inhibiting tumors in mice than a common anti-cancer drug.[21]

More tests

Jerry McLaughlin, along with doctoral student Nicholas Ober-lies, continued to study and test paw paw at Purdue, throughout the latter 1990's. They published two scientific articles in 1997 on the effectiveness of paw paw in killing cancer cells that are resistant to anticancer agents. Their findings were that paw paw had a special affinity for these multiple drug resistant (MDR) cells.

McLaughlin was quoted in the *Purdue News* explaining this phenomenon:

> "Multidrug-resistant cancer is hard to treat because the cancer cell has developed a mechanism to get around the anti-cancer agent. . . . Tumor cells that survive chemotherapy treatments often recover with increased resistance to the agent used in the original treatment program as well as to other related drugs."[22]

As I noted earlier, MDR cells typically have the ability to produce a "pump" mechanism that literally pushes anti-cancer agents such as chemotherapy drugs out of the cells.[23] The chemo gets into the cell, but the cell responds with "Sorry, not interested," and kicks the chemo out the door. Potentially any cell, cancerous or normal, can produce these pumps. But normal cells hardly ever produce them and only a very few cancer cells produce them. But it is these *few cancer cells* that remain *resistant* to chemotherapy drugs, and consequently are the cells that multiply and *cause cancer to return.*

What McLaughlin and his associates discovered was that paw paw, because it attacks the ability of a cell to produce energy, starves these MDR cells of the energy needed to use their own pumps. What is evident, then, is that paw paw's deadly effect on the energy-producing mitochondria has a two-prong effect. It kills regular cancer cells by depriving them of energy necessary to survive, and it helps chemotherapy drugs to kill resistant cells by depriving them of the energy needed to reject the chemo!

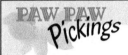

Tale of Three Cities

There are three U.S. cities named "Paw Paw." Geographically, they span quite a bit of territory!

Paw Paw, West Virginia

Paw Paw, Michigan

Paw Paw, Illinois

Studies on humans

Before making paw paw available on the general market, Dr. McLaughlin, Gina B. Benson, and James Forsythe M.D. conducted an extensive study in conjunction with Cancer Screening and Treatment Center of Nevada.[24] 94 volunteer participants were recruited, including 20 terminal cases. All the subjects had been diagnosed with clinical cancer. Some were undergoing chemotherapy and/or radiation. A variety of tumor types were represented.

The study preceded the first marketing of paw paw to the public in 2003. Obviously, the body of knowledge of paw paw as well as the treatment of cancer in general has grown since then. But this early study is quite fascinating and instructive even today.

A standardized extract of paw paw was used throughout. The paw paw capsules each contained 12.5 milligrams of the extract. It was found that one capsule, taken four times a day with food, was tolerable, avoiding nausea and vomiting. It was determined that there were no ill effects on the liver or bone marrow. In fact, little or no adverse side effects of any kind were noted.

Preliminary studies included three volunteers with terminal ovarian cancers. Ovarian cancers are rated by a test that measures the level of CA-125 (Cancer Antigen 125) in the blood. Within one week the CA-125 levels of one patient were reduced by 66%!

The study continued over a period of 1 ½ years. New patients were added during this period. As the study progressed, results looked more and more promising. The study was titled *A novel mechanism for the control of clinical cancer. Inhibition of the productions of adenosine triphosphate (ATP) with*

a standardized extract off paw paw (asimina triloba, Annonaceae).
Here are descriptions of ten sample cases, excerpted from the
study. They typify the general results of the overall study. . . .

Patient's breast cancer is contained:

> Participant #1 is a 53 year old female. She was diag-
> nosed with breast cancer in 1996, and underwent a
> lumpectomy and radiation treatments. In January,
> 2000 the cancer returned to the bone. Further radia-
> tion treatments were performed to the right hip and
> spine area concluding in 2002. Alkaline phosphatase
> was measured in the blood as a way to monitor the
> progress of the disease. The normal range is 0-136,
> and those with cancer of the bone have elevated lev-
> els. The blood test taken in September 2002 was at
> 327. She started taking four Paw Paw capsules per
> day in November. By December the levels slightly
> decreased to 242. In February 2003 the alkaline phos-
> phatase level decreased to 144. Since February the
> levels have remained stable (between 144 and 150).
> According to her physician, since the levels are re-
> maining stable it shows that the cancer is contained
> and not doing further damage to the bone. She re-
> ports that she has more energy and stamina when
> taking the Paw Paw capsules.

Man with bone cancer decreases tumor size taking
paw paw alone:

> Participant #2 is a 63 year old male with a bone tu-
> mor in the neck. On July 30, 2002, the bone tumor
> which showed up on the x-ray was measured as a
> 7rnrn cavity with a 5rnrn mass on the neck. He did

not undergo any other treatments besides the Paw Paw capsules. He started taking the Paw Paw capsules in September 2002. Another x-ray taken on March 13, 2003 showed a significant decrease of the tumor size: the cavity was measured to be 4.5rnrn with a 3rnrn mass.

Woman with breast cancer improves "remarkably":

Participant #13 is a 52 year old female with breast cancer. She has not undergone any conventional treatments since being diagnosed. She has taken the Paw Paw capsules since October 2002. She reports that the pain in the breast has decreased and the non-cancerous fibrocystic lumps have reduced in size. Her doctor reports she has been doing "remarkably well" considering that she has not had surgery, chemotherapy, or radiation. She says that she feels good and also has had some weight gain.

Woman with breast cancer had no surgery or chemotherapy, tumor reduced:

Participant #14 is 59 year old female with breast cancer. She has not had any surgery, chemotherapy, or radiation treatments. She started taking four capsules of Paw Paw in November 2002. The blood tests for the breast cancer tumor markers (CA 27-29) were consistent from 9/12/02 to 12/3/02 with both being 24.6. In March 2003 all the blood tests were within normal range. The tumor size has also reduced.

Woman with breast cancer takes paw paw concurrently with chemotherapy, achieves complete remission:

> Participant #15 is 62 year old female with breast cancer. She decided to undergo chemotherapy treatments and take the Paw Paw capsules concurrently. The chemotherapy treatments lasted seven months. The tumor almost completely disappeared, as evidenced by magnetic resonance imaging and ultrasound. She decided to undergo surgery as well to remove any traces of the cancer. Removal of 14 axillary lymph nodes showed no metastatic cancer. This was followed by radiation. Her most recent screen showed no cancer in the breast. She is in complete remission and believed to be cancer free.

Woman with Stage Four breast cancer significantly improved, stabilized:

> Participant #20 is 70 year old female with stage four breast cancer. Within just six weeks of taking the Paw Paw capsules she saw a 50% percent reduction in the CA 27-29 tumor markers, which went from 160 to 80. The size of the tumor was also reduced significantly. Since she had not changed any other treatment protocol, her physician is convinced that the Paw Paw is responsible for her improvement and stabilization.

Man with Stage Four lung cancer overcomes resistant cancer cells:

> Participant #42 is a 66 year old male with stage four lung cancer. He previously had undergone two years

of chemotherapy, but the lung cancer had become resistant. Within two months of taking the Paw Paw capsules his CEA tumor markers decreased from 275 to 222. He also had a weight gain of 5 pounds and experienced no side effects to the Paw Paw capsules. Previous to taking the Paw Paw capsules he was bedridden or was in a wheelchair. His health improved to the point that he is now able to walk on his own.

Man deemed terminal with inoperable Stage Four melanoma regains energy, resumes normal activities:

Participant #51 is a 60 year old male diagnosed with stage four melanoma which had metastasized from his arm to the lungs and lymph nodes. The doctors could not operate to remove the lung mass. The tumor started causing difficulty in breathing and he was expected to expire in February 2003. Since starting the Paw Paw in November 2002 he had an easier time breathing within a few days, and he has been feeling much better. He also has been able to get out of bed and even progressed to riding a bike, walking uphill, and working on his farm. Interestingly, two fatty tumors on his arm have also decreased considerably in size. He also reports that the toe nail fungus he has had for 10 years is clearing up.

Man with prostate cancer markedly improves:

Participant #64 is a 56 year old male diagnosed with prostate cancer. The cancer was confirmed by biopsy. He started taking four Paw Paw capsules per day in

October 2002. His PSA[25] levels dropped to 2.08 on
12/23/02 down from a PSA of 3.85 taken two months
previously and continued to take the Paw Paw capsules until April 2003.

Man with Stage Four prostate cancer reduces tumors:.

Participant #84 is a 73 year old male with stage four
prostate cancer which had spread to other parts (left
neck, abdomen, and hip bone) of the body. Within six
weeks of taking the Paw Paw the CT scan showed a
25 % reduction in the tumor masses. His PSA levels
are remaining constant.

The study summarizes the use of paw paw along with chemotherapy:

Due to the positive responses from the aforementioned case studies and from many of the original 94
participants, it is apparent that the paw paw extracts
are an effective supplement for the regulation of cancers of various types. It also looks as if the extracts
are an effective adjunct to chemotherapeutic agents.
When taken with chemotherapy, in some instances,
the patients and physicians noticed an above average
amount of tumor shrinkage after the first treatments
than would normally be expected with chemotherapy alone. The synergistic benefit may be attributed
to the novel action of the acetogenins causing ATP
depletion resulting in apoptosis of the cancer cells.
Chemotherapy resistance, with ATP-driven efflux
pumps, is also thwarted by the ATP-depleting action
of the acetogenins resulting in renewed cellular ac-

cumulation of the chemotherapeutic agent. *Thus, the combination of chemotherapy, which also induces apoptosis, and paw paw extracts had an increased effect.* [Emphasis added]

Summary of paw paw used as the sole treatment:

. . . Paw paw extracts have been effective, by both objective and subjective measurements, even when they are not combined with chemotherapy or radiation. Many participants have enjoyed an extended longevity and also have improved their quality of life with this supplement. Those that were weakened or bedridden now have more energy to do those things that they enjoy. Others that have been given only a couple of months to live have surpassed the doctors' predictions in a marvelous way. Even more promising are those that have decreased the size of the tumors without the loss of hair, nausea, bone marrow depression, induction of new cancers, or other side effects.

The report concludes the following. If you read only one paragraph of this book, read this:

The paw paw extract is unlike drugs because it is a complex mixture of natural compounds rather than a single entity. This represents a new approach in the alleviation of clinical cancer. Paw paw is an herbal supplement product with clinical effectiveness but with a very low toxicity. Paw paw has a unique mode of action focusing on depleting the energy-producing molecule ATP. Rather than poisoning the

DNA as with most chemotherapy, paw paw is able to exploit a previously neglected biochemical difference, i.e., the voracious uptake of glucose, in cancer cells versus normal cells. . . . It is now apparent that mitochondrial inhibition (ATP depletion) offers a novel mechanism for the control of clinical cancer.

—○—

Since the above study, thousands of other cancer patients have benefited from paw paw. Although documentation on these cases is sparse, anecdotal reports do appear now and again. One natural health practitioner noted for her work with paw paw is Lorene Benoit, MHH, CHC, CRA who practices in Canada. She notes several of her clients and how they have benefited from paw paw:[26]

- A 75 year old female contracts Non Hodgkin's Lymphoma in 2002. She undergoes conventional treatments for years, but her condition worsens. She finally starts on paw paw in July 2010 and by the following October her tumors are gone.
- Male client diagnosed with lung cancer rejects chemotherapy. After a paw paw sequence he is cancer-free.
- A 17 year old male diagnosed with brain cancer, and on a paw paw regimen, at the time of Benoit's report had been alive two years longer than doctors expected.
- Male with leukemia (cancer of the blood) has severe reactions to chemotherapy, begins high-dose paw paw program. Within 2 weeks his blood count is normal, doctor no longer recommends chemo.

- Male with colon cancer has tumor removed surgically but malignant lymph nodes remain. He rejects chemotherapy in favor of paw paw program in October, 2007. By March, 2008 he is cancer-free.

In short, again and again paw paw has shown that it can be extremely effective in slowing, halting, and eradicating cancers of all types. Data suggests that paw paw can be especially effective when used *concurrently* with traditional treatments. Let's talk about that next. . . .

6. Can Paw Paw Be Used Along With Chemotherapy and Radiation?

Paw paw and chemotherapy

I've always believed, as do many others, in the "shotgun" approach to cancer. "What is the *shotgun approach*?" you may ask. To wildly mix a metaphor, the shotgun approach is simply not putting all your eggs in one basket. A shotgun doesn't shoot a single bullet, but sprays many bits of ammunition at the target.

While the subject of this book is nominally treating cancer with paw paw, it's not to be inferred that using *only* paw paw is the intention.

Paw paw extract is distinctly different from typical chemotherapy drugs. Chemotherapy drugs are relatively simple in their chemistry compared to paw paw — which is a natural combination of many compounds. Most synthesized drugs in the pharmaceutical world are designed to act upon only one target (*i.e.* cellular receptor, gene, protein, etc.). Cancer, however, can be the result of many thousands of complex targets. The fact that cancer is so complex has been a major stumbling block in finding a single cure.[27] Paw paw can be effective against so many types of cancer because of its very complexity—an array of more than over 50 recognized acetogenin compounds, each working in its own way.[28] You might say that paw paw *all by itself* is a shotgun approach!

Chemotherapy generally works more quickly than paw paw, but chemo alone is definitely not to be considered generally more effective than paw paw.[29] *No* treatment works the same way or equally well on different patients. Sometimes a certain chemo drug will work well on one person and not so well on another patient with a similar diagnosis. Keep in mind that chemotherapy alone has a stunningly poor rate of curing cancer. One study,[30] involving patients in the United States and Australia, found that the "cure" rate for chemotherapy (defined as survival for five years after diagnosis or first treatment) was—are your ready?—*barely over two percent!* It's estimated that the cure rate for *alternative* treatments in general is much, much higher.

Statistics, though, are overall averages—not guarantees. Paw paw, just like any other treatment, may benefit one individual more than another. Hence the wisdom of the shotgun approach. This does not mean one should indiscriminately throw everything you've got at the cancer. Many remedies conflict with each other; they could cancel each other out or produce unwanted outcomes. Combining various treatments requires an intelligent approach. They must *complement* each other, not *conflict* with each other. (In Chapter 9 we'll get into more detail about which supplements might be beneficial when taken with paw paw and which supplements might be detrimental.)

Chemotherapy and paw paw do not appear to conflict with each other. Experience has shown that patients experience no ill effects from taking both during the same time-

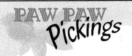

Paw Paw's Unique Ability

There is no pharma-ceutical in the whole of standard medicine that kills multiple drug re-sistant cancer cells the way paw paw's aceto-genins do. Some che-motherapy regimens used <u>alone</u> can actu-ally be carcinogenic and <u>create</u> cells that chemotherapy cannot then destroy!

frame.[31] Further, studies have indicated that in many cases patients given chemo and paw paw did exceptionally well—better than most that were given chemo only.

As noted earlier, paw paw goes after those multiple drug resistant (MDR) cells that chemo leaves be-hind, and this can make all the difference.

Bottom line: If you decide on chemotherapy you should strongly consider taking paw paw as well. And for those who experience intoler-able side effects from chemo—and therefore reject it—they should definitely consider taking paw paw alone. As I said previously, it works more slowly than chemo, but it has a strong record of killing cancer cells, and has virtually no side effects when properly taken.

Paw paw and radiation treatment

There are several types of radiation used in treating cancer. The type selected for a particular patient will depend on many factors—the type, extent and size of the tumor(s), the location of the cancer in the body, the age and health of the patient, etc. Radiation therapy consists of a high-energy radiation source directed from outside the body or from implantation of radioactive material inside the body.[32]

Radiation works by damaging the DNA of the cancer cells. It can also damage normal cells, just as chemotherapy can — so side effects are common.

Should paw paw be considered as an additional treatment alongside radiation? Well, certainly yes if the patient is *also* receiving chemotherapy. In this case paw paw will function as it would with chemo alone, helping to rid the body of resistant cells as well as killing regular cancer cells.

But what about using paw paw when radiation is the only therapy being employed? Certainly, paw paw will not interfere in any appreciable way with radiation. It's like asking the question "If the enemy soldiers are being bombed, would it hurt to use artillery fire as well?" It's rather analogous to using chemotherapy alongside radiation — attacking the cancer on two fronts.

If a tumor has not metastasized, sometimes highly targeted radiation is used in lieu of removal of the tumor by surgery. But the question may linger: "Did it get *all* the cancer?" Paw paw in such cases can be an insurance policy, assuring that any residual cancer is being attacked without resorting to chemotherapy and its attendant side effects.

In my wife's case, the chemo/paw paw combination had reduced her tumors to the point where surgery was considered. But because she was not deemed a good candidate for surgery, targeted radiation treatments were given instead. She continued to take paw paw alongside the radiation. When the radiation was discontinued due to adverse side effects, we kept her on paw paw for several months afterwards and achieved remission.

I think the final word on the question is that paw paw, not being effectively toxic and having no significant side effects, is not detrimental when taken alongside radiation therapy. Even though it might turn out that radiation alone might have done the total job without needing outside help, as far as paw paw goes—*it couldn't hurt.* But do observe the recommendation that paw paw *not* be taken when *no* cancer is present (see Chapter 8). The exception to this might be to take paw paw for a limited time after remission is achieved, as a preventive against the return of the cancer. (More about this on Page 64.)

What about paw paw with surgery?

There are many types of surgery which might be used in the course of cancer treatment.[33] Typically when "curative" surgery is used a patient's cancer has not metastasized. The cancer is simply cut out of the body. After surgery the removed tumor is usually analyzed to make sure that *all* the cancer was removed. The patient may also be subsequently scanned for any possible remaining cancer in the body.

If the surgery is declared completely successful and the patient cancer-free, there is obviously no need for further treatment, and this would include paw paw. This would be a time to go from treatment mode into prevention mode, following healthy guidelines and taking cancer preventing supplements, such as Curcumin, Alpha Lipoic Acid, fish oil, etc. I would advise researching healthy diets and cancer-preventing foods and supplements—outside the topic of this book.

However, the result is not always that definitive. If there is any doubt about remaining cancer in the body, it wouldn't hurt to continue taking the paw paw for a while. Again, just be sure the paw paw is not taken for any significant period when there is *no* cancer.

—o—

Some patients seeking advice on natural, non-pharmaceutical supplements and treatments may want to consult with a specialist to help them create a personalized program. Let's look into that next. . . .

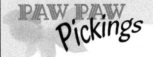

Growing a Paw Paw Tree?

Although paw paw is a forest "understory" tree in the wild, when cultivated it needs full-sun exposure in order to have good fruit production. Look for a planting site that doesn't get wind, which is harmful to a paw paw's large leaves. If you will plant a seedling, locate a site for it in full sun, but protect it from full sunlight for the first two years with shade cloth or tree shelters. The best soil for paw paw is slightly acidic, fertile, moist, deep, and well-drained. Avoid planting the tree in an area with wet, heavy, or alkaline soil.

Read more :

http://www.ehow.com/how_590131
2_plant-paw-paw-tree.html

7. Will I Need to Consult a Natural Health Practioner or Alternative Physician if I Take Paw Paw?

Coordinating with your oncologist

First, it's always a good idea to let your oncologist in on *any* treatment you are undertaking. Chances are, he/she won't be familiar with paw paw. And that's OK—most oncologists aren't into natural remedies. I do think, though, that you will find your oncologist supportive of any sincere endeavor you are making to take charge of your own treatment—and they'll at least appreciate the fact that you're keeping them informed.

On the other hand, if your oncologist is dead set against natural treatments, then you have a problem. You may want to consider changing to another oncologist rather than taking paw paw (or anything else not officially prescribed) behind their back.

Defining natural and alternative practices

The area of non-conventional medicine can be confusing. Sometimes the terms overlap; some are licensed MDs while others are licensed under other banners. You will see some practitioners listed as "alternative," "complementary," "naturopathic," and "homeopathic," etc.

There are licensed MDs who also practice Complementary or Alternative medicine. Others are licensed as "naturopaths," and carry the "ND" (Naturopathic Doctor) label. Let's rule out homeopathic doctors here—homeopathy is an entirely separate kind of medicine that deals in very small quantities of drugs, typically a highly diluted version of the disease being treated. This has nothing to do with natural medicines such as paw paw.

You might find a practitioner that could help you with paw paw among licensed MD's who practice Complementary (or Alternative) Medicine, or among Naturopathic Practitioners.

Finding a natural practitioner

What is a naturopathic doctor (ND)? Naturopathic physicians are trained, licensed professionals. Currently 16 states license naturopathic doctors, although they are not "MDs." Applicants to accredited naturopathic colleges must have bachelor degrees, and must have prerequisites just like applicants to conventional medical schools.[34] Don't think that they simply read a few books and hang up a shingle.

Naturopathic physicians typically work *together* with conventional doctors. They deal with advice about dietary matters and pharmaceuticals, as well as many matters for which they have been trained. You may decide that you don't really need a naturopath, or indeed live in an area that does not license them. Expect that not all naturopaths are familiar with paw paw.

Do you absolutely need to consult this type of professional if you are taking paw paw? No. We're not dealing with a highly toxic drug here, or something that might conflict with conventional treatments. And there is no legal requirement that you take any natural product under professional supervision. But many might feel more comfortable in the hands of an experienced natural practitioner.

The best way to locate a naturopath is through their professional association, AANP (American Association of Naturopathic Physicians). There is a searchable directory on their website.[35]

The decision to use a practitioner of non-conventional medicine is really a personal one. If you have an interest in or curiosity about various treatments outside the realm of standard medicine, then by all means follow your instincts. Some may feel uncomfortable taking *anything* not prescribed ("over-the-counter").

Others are used to doing their own research and feel they don't need any help in making these types of decisions.

The choice is yours. Just remember that paw paw, while certainly a strong medicine, is not very likely to conflict with any standard treatment or give you any appreciable side effects. If you've read and understood what's in this book, you are certainly prepared enough to self-administer paw paw!

8. Where Do I Get It and How Much Should I Take?

The matter of dosage is important. First though, let's talk about exactly what paw paw product to take. The situation is different from typical supplements manufactured by this brand and that, all variations on the same product. Dr. McLaughlin has published his process of harvesting, extracting, and standardization, and has worked with only one company to produce and sell the resulting product. He receives no financial rewards for his work.

If there were many reliable sources I would list them, but in the case of paw paw there is only one, namely Nature's Sunshine, a well-established company that produces a variety of health related supplements. There are other paw paw products, but they do not come with the reliability and standardization found in the *Nature's Sunshine* product.

I know it must sound like I'm advertising for a single company—I'm not. As stated in the disclaimer in the beginning of this book, I have absolutely no financial interest in selling any brand of paw paw to anyone. If there were other reliable sources with a standardized product I would list them—there simply aren't any.

Where can I get paw paw?

You probably won't find paw paw at your local pharmacy or vitamin shop. Your best bet, perhaps your only bet, is to purchase it online—or by phone order. The name of the product is *Paw Paw Cell-Reg*. *Nature's Sunshine* has a sister website at *HealthySunshine.com* with a page dedicated to paw paw alone, where you can read about and order the product:

http://www.healthy-sunshine.com/paw-paw-cell-reg

(If you prefer to order by telephone, you can call Healthy Sunshine in the United States at 888-523-1727.) You will see that paw paw is sold in bottles of 180 capsules. Expect to pay $40-$45 per bottle. The bottles will come marked with a lot number and a date through which full potency will be present. Since one bottle is pretty close to a month's supply for most patients, this is quite a bargain I'd say.

How much do I take?

So now the paw paw arrives, and you want to know how much to take and when to take it. The recommended dosage on the bottle may specify 2 capsules 3 times daily (6 capsules per day). Note that once in a while the harvest of the twigs may yield a paw paw crop with a variance in strength of the acetogenins. Should this occur, a slightly different dosage may be recommended.

But, as in many things, one size does not fit all. There is a way to determine the perfect dose for you as an individual. You might recall that paw paw can produce nausea if one takes too much (even when taken with food). You may want to use the following method. It's a plan for determining your dosage, while gradually "breaking in" your body's tolerance of the medicine. . . .

- On Day 1 take 1 capsule with your lunch and 1 capsule with dinner.
- On Day 2, take 2 capsules with lunch and 1 at dinner.
- On Day 3, take 2 at lunch and 2 at dinner.
- On Day 4, take 1 at breakfast, 2 at lunch, and 2 at dinner.
- On Day 6, take 2 at breakfast, 2 at lunch, and 2 at dinner.

So, as you can see, each day you are increasing your total dose for the day by one capsule. Do this until you reach a dosage that produces nausea. At this point *cut back* by one capsule. That is your dose—the maximum you can take without experiencing nausea. (See more about dosage on Page 90.)

I have heard of some brave souls who slowly increased to over 20 capsules per day, by very gradually increasing over a long period—several weeks. This is extreme, of course, but some have done it nevertheless.

What about dosages for children?

For children's dosages it will require a little math. Assuming the average adult is 200 pounds, and the average adult dosage is 6 capsules per day (2 capsules three times per day at meals), a child's dosage could be determined by their weight. If the child weighed 100 pounds, that would come out to three capsules (one half the adult dosage). A child weighing 50 lbs would be given one and one-half capsules per day, (one quarter the adult dosage) etc.

Remember that capsules can be opened and their contents be mixed into a little applesauce (for example). This would work well, since taking paw paw with food is desirable. (See Dr. McLaughlin's recommendation on Page 91.)

What should *not be* taken when taking paw paw?

Well, firstly, don't take anything *with* paw paw that you wouldn't take by itself—*without* paw paw. Try to avoid any food or supplement that tends to make you nauseous, especially when first starting with paw paw. Other than that, there is nothing that's especially problematic to take concurrently with paw paw. If you're in doubt about taking prescription meds ask the prescriber if there's any contra-indication. Chances are most medicines will be OK. One source I have seen claims that it is not advisable to take paw paw with nutritional supplements like CoQ10 and thyroid stimulators, as these supplements enhance mitochondrial complex 1 activities and energy production, respectively.[36] Since paw paw is trying to diminish mitochondrial activity and CoQ10 and similar products are trying to *activate* mitochondrial activity it might seem logical that they shouldn't be taken concurrently. But studies have shown differently. No problems were seen with taking antioxidant and thyroid products alongside paw paw.

In the next chapter, we'll talk about enzymes, and how not to take them at the same *time of day* that you are taking paw paw. If you take vitamins, there would be no need to stop them.

Should paw paw be taken as a cancer preventative?

Taking paw paw for a short time will generally do you no harm whether you have cancer or not. But if you do *not* currently have cancer it may not be the wisest thing to take paw paw as a cancer preventative. Remember that prolonged use can be detrimental to normal cells. With no cancer cells to attract the acetogenins in paw paw they will seek out other cells, particularly the faster growing, energy-consuming ones. These would include cells in the digestive tract and intestines, for example.

Paw paw is sometimes used for conditions other than cancer. It has been known, for instance, to cure toenail fungus. (Yes, really!) But it is not recommended for prolonged use. Don't take paw paw for more than a month or so if you don't have cancer.

Sometimes a remission of the cancer may be achieved, but it leaves you

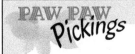

How Successful is Chemotherapy?

The average five-year-survival rate attributable to chemotherapy in adult patients with all types of cancers, according to a 2004 scientific study, is 2.1%

Graeme Morgan, Robyn Ward, Michael Barton *The Contribution of Cytotoxic Chemotherapy to 5-year Survival in Adult Malignancies*, 2004.

with a question: Should you continue the paw paw to prevent the cancer from returning? The answer is yes—but only for six months after remission. Dr. McLaughlin recommends in these cases that after the first six months the patient take full doses of paw paw for one month, then nothing for the second month. Then back to a full dose for the third month, etc., alternating on and off months.[37]

Sometimes, after remission, nodules or unidentified anomalies subsequently show up on a scan. The oncologist may not be sure if there is malignancy or not, and recommend monitoring for awhile, to see if there's growth in the suspicious areas. "Monitoring" usually means having the area scanned every three months or so. In this case you might take paw paw "just in case." But, again, don't prolong the use past 6 months if no cancer is present.

What should I tell my doctor about my taking paw paw?

If you are undergoing conventional treatment while also taking paw paw it would be a good idea to make a list of *all* the supplements and alternative medicines you are taking and give a copy to your oncologist. A significant part of cancer treatment is evaluating the effectiveness of the treatment as you go along. Your cancer will be regularly measured and your progress noted, alongside the specifics of the treatment you are receiving. Chances are that your oncologist will find that your progress is better than was expected. This is because conventional doctors know very little about the effectiveness of paw paw. It's simply not in their vocabulary, and it's not expected to be.

If your doctor sees unusual progress, and isn't aware of your paw paw regimen, your progress will certainly be attributed to whatever standard treatment you are being given, or you will be deemed exceptionally receptive to treatment.

At least, if the doctor is *aware* of your "extra-curricular" treatments he might suspect that they have something to do with why you're doing as well as you are.

My wife's oncologist was made aware of her non-conventional treatment, mainly the paw paw. He was not specifically all that interested in alternative methods, but, noting Josée's exceptional progress, repeatedly told us "Keep doing whatever you're doing."

I have heard of some cancer patients who took paw paw and did so remarkably well that the doctor wondered if the patient had been misdiagnosed in the first place. (It's my understanding that this is not uncommon.) In fact, this happened with Josée. The oncologist wondered if she had been misdiagnosed as having Stage IV lung cancer. Perhaps there had been a mistake. But, early on in the process Josée had switched from one hospital's cancer center to another hospital's cancer facility.

We reminded the second doctor that the diagnosis arrived at in the first hospital— entirely independent from the second—had been identical, also Stage IV lung cancer. The chances of both facilities making the same wrong diagnosis were very small indeed. I do believe his mind received a special ray of light at that moment—he was a thoughtful and perceptive fellow. And, though he never pursued paw paw in any substantial way, he remained open-minded throughout our relationship.

What are the side effects of paw paw?

There are reportedly no serious side effects. Of course, as in any medication not everyone will be affected in the same way. But in the clinical studies of paw paw no substantial side effects were reported. If you are experiencing nausea and are sure it's being caused by the paw paw, you're probably taking too much paw paw. Lower your dosage. You might want to go back to just one capsule per day for a few days, and then gradually increase.

As mentioned earlier, if you take paw paw when cancer is absent, you risk damaging normal cells in the body. (See Page 64 about taking paw paw as a preventative.)

If you are undergoing standard treatments, such as chemotherapy or radiation, and are experiencing side effects, they are probably a result of those treatments, not the paw paw. I did once hear a warning from a naturopath that "paw paw can damage the liver"—but I haven't been able to find any reports that would validate that. I can say from personal experience that my wife took paw paw steadily for the better part of a year and her liver is just fine.

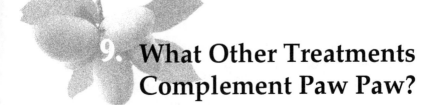

9. What Other Treatments Complement Paw Paw?

If you're planning on taking more than two or three supplements to help fight your cancer, you might want to consult with a natural practitioner (*See* Chapter 7). Planning your supplements involves making some judicious choices and a good knowledge of what's out there, what's promising, and what's doable. You may want to investigate the many books written about cancer and healthy foods and supplements.

There is only one book I'm aware of that covers supplements in general as well as paw paw in particular. That is *The Paw Paw Program: A Christopher Columbus Approach to Cancer...* by Lorene Benoit. Ms. Benoit, a Certified Herbal Consultant who lives in Canada, covers everything from supplements to diet to exercise to recipes for preparing healthy meals.

The following suggestions are specifically aimed at patients who have decided to take paw paw, whether alongside standard treatments, or in lieu of standard treatments. . . .

How do protease enzymes help paw paw to work better?

What's an enzyme anyway? And what does "protease" mean? Here's a definition from Wikipedia:

> A protease (also called peptidase or proteinase) is any enzyme that performs proteolysis, that is, begins

protein catabolism[38] by hydrolysis of the peptide bonds that link amino acids together in the polypeptide chain forming the protein. Proteases have evolved multiple times, and different classes of protease can perform the same reaction by completely different catalytic mechanisms. Proteases can be found in animals, plants, bacteria, archaea, and viruses.

Well, that's a lot of big words there! All you really have to know here is that protease enzymes break up proteins in foods in the digestion process. They also can break up the tough outer "shell" of cancer cells. This helps the acetogenins in paw paw penetrate the affected cells.

But the obvious question arises: Will the enzymes be used up in the digestive process and never get into the bloodstream and be delivered to the cells? This obvious question has an obvious answer: Take the enzymes on an empty stomach. First thing in the morning? Late afternoon? Before going to bed? Not so hard to figure out.

The next question is: What *kind* of protease enzymes should you take? The potency of protease is measured in "HUT" (Hemoglobin Unit Tyrosine) units. The accepted standard is set by the Food Chemical Codex (FCC), which operates under the Federal Drug Administration. The higher the HUT, the more powerful the protease in the supplement. So if you compare two different brands having *equal weight* (mg), and the HUT of Brand A is twice that of Brand B that would indicate that Brand A has twice the strength of Brand B. Typically, the HUT number can range from 25,000 to 375,000. Author and herbal consultant Lorene Benoit recommends a protease enzyme that is rated at 60,000 HUT or higher.[39] I wouldn't accept one with an HUT lower than that. Be careful in selecting an enzyme product. If you don't see the HUT number on the label there's no way to tell how potent it is.

What about antioxidants? Should I take them while taking paw paw?

There are so many benefits from antioxidant supplements that they must always be seriously considered—whether one has cancer or not. Oxidation is a very common phenomenon. When you see an apple slice turn brown, you are witnessing oxidation. Oxygen reacts with the apple and turns it brown.

Oxidation is a natural process, and it happens inside the body as well. Nature has provided—in many of the foods we eat—antioxidants to defend against the negative effects of oxidation in our bodies. However, nature doesn't always totally succeed in clearing the body of damaged cells. The result is the creation of "free radicals." These are atoms that have an extra charge—and they can do a lot of harm. Free radicals can damage the DNA, resulting in the creation of cancerous cells.[40]

It's obvious, then, that antioxidants are extremely important in maintaining health. It's beyond the scope of this book to go into all the foods and their value as antioxidants. But certain foods can be mentioned as having high antioxidant properties. These include fresh fruits and vegetables, legumes and nuts.

One handy way to prepare these foods is to make an antioxidant "cocktail" in a blender, *NutriBullet (Magic Bullet)*, or similar machine. You can (as an example) put in some fresh greens—such as raw kale, spinach, or broccoli—add some fresh fruit (pear, banana, etc.) throw in some raw almonds and some blueberries. Add a dash of turmeric (curcumin), some ground cloves, and cinnamon. Add water and blend until smooth. Now *there* is a dose of antioxidants!

But, in addition to eating healthy foods, supplements can provide even greater concentrations of anti-oxidants. Alpha Lipoic Acid would be a good example. We'll talk about mangosteen juice/extract below.

Can you take antioxidant supplements concurrently with paw paw? Yes; feel free—they won't interfere with paw paw's action.

What's all this about Mangosteen?

The mangosteen (not related to the mango) is a fruit that grows in places like China and the Philippines. Products based on this fruit seemed to burst onto the market around 2002, and mangosteen has gained wide popularity as a supplement for all kinds of ailments and conditions. There is mangosteen juice sold in bottles, and mangosteen "blends" of all sorts. There are also mangosteen capsules, extracts, etc.—all widely available.

The question is, is it all hype or does mangosteen have actual value? Well, there is a lot of hype, and, yes, there is evidence that mangosteen products have value. The key compounds found in mangosteen are called "xanthones," and these have antioxidant, antibacterial, antifungal, anti-inflammatory, and antitumor qualities.[41] Yes, you read that right. Mangosteen has been used in folk medicine for thousands of years. People have used it to treat mucus, cystitis, diarrhea, dysentery, fever, gonorrhea, and stomatosis—as well as skin disorders such as eczema and pruritus.

Does it help, and is it safe to take mangosteen concurrently with paw paw? Because mangosteen is such a strong antioxidant there was originally some question about its use with paw paw. The theory went that, since paw paw is trying to *lower* ATP levels, while antioxidants *raise* ATP levels, the two would conflict, canceling each other out. But this opinion is generally no longer held. A study by the Ford Cancer Clinic showed that a mangosteen blend did not diminish the effect of paw paw, and in fact enhanced it.[42]

So go ahead with it if you so choose. Mangosteen comes several ways: the pure juice or mangosteen juice blended with other juices—sold in bottles, freeze-dried and sun-dried versions sold in capsules and what-not. Some products are made from the entire fruit, some from the rind (pericarp) only, some from the juice only, and various combinations of these. Keep in mind that most of the xanthones in mangosteen are in the *rind*. One capsule version on the market contains extract from the pericarp only.

Bottom line on using mangosteen with paw paw— recommended.

How about Noni juice?

The benefits of Noni juice were brought to public attention in the 1990's by Neil Solomon MD, PhD. The juice of the tropical Noni fruit has been used medicinally for centuries by natives of Polynesia, particularly Tahiti. Solomon wrote several books on the topic, and many people claim to have greatly benefited from the juice, particularly cancer patients. Solomon demonstrated Noni's ability to kill cancer cells in laboratory animals.[43]

I have personal experience with Noni. Our dog, the aforementioned Sparky, drank an ounce of Noni every day during his treatment for non-Hodgkin's lymphoma. We credit his miraculous survival to an excellent veterinary oncologist and Noni juice. Noni does not have a pleasant taste; in fact it reminds me somewhat of prune juice that has gone rancid. But you can get used to gulping down an ounce or two, and alternately it can be mixed with other fruit juices to make it more palatable.

If you decide to use Noni, you want to buy the pure Noni juice—Noni being the sole ingredient. The kind we favor is undiluted and comes in glass bottles. There are several brands. The one we used is Tahitian Noni from *Tahiti Naturel*,[44] a reliable product available mainly by mail order in the United States.

So, you're asking, how does Noni get along with paw paw? The answer is "fine." There have been no reported problems concerning taking the two concurrently. Note: You will see later that paw paw should be taken with meals. Noni works best when taken on an empty stomach. (First thing in the morning would work well.)

Etc., etc. . . .

There are basically two kinds of alternative supplements. The first kind includes products and natural substances that actually *kill* cancer cells ("cytotoxins"). The second kind includes nutrients and products that promote good health and help the immune system itself to better destroy the cancer cells.

There are many, many foods and products that are cited and marketed to do the latter (as well as helping to *prevent* cancer)—healthy foods, vitamins, and supplements. These have been well-documented, and there are many books and online sources providing this information. My goodness, one could write a book on anti-oxidants alone—there are so many. This wide category of cancer fighters is beyond the range of this book, but that is not to say that I don't encourage you to investigate them. One particular book that I recommend, because of its regarding of these supplements and foods in relation to *paw paw* is Lorene Benoit's book *The Paw Paw Program*.[45]

Getting back to the first category, here are some natural (plant based) products which can be considered cancer treatments:

- Beta Glucan
- Ellagic Acid
- Emulsified Vitamin A
- Essiac Tea
- Graviola
- Laetrile B-17
- MGN-3
- Papaya Leaves (N.B. The papaya is called "paw paw' in some countries—such as Australia—*but is not related to the American Paw Paw!*)
- Paw Paw
- Vitamin C (intravenous, high dosages)

Of all of these, paw paw has been rated the most effective by reliable sources. One such source I would highly recommend that you visit online is:

www.alternativecancer.us

This is a comprehensive alternative cancer site that has no fi-

nancial ties with any of the products it lists. I found it refresh-
ingly objective and helpful.

For further exploration, here is a list of strictly *herbal*
remedies that have been used to fight cancer. Herbs are defined as plants that don't develop a woody stem (as trees or
bushes do). I've included a brief note with each, referring to
some of the types of cancer each has been associated with
(*though not limited to*). For more information, check out

*http://www.canceractive.com/cancer-active-page-
link.aspx?n=3054* .

I would strongly recommend researching any of these
you are considering using. There are such matters as dosage
and side effects to be considered. This list is merely to suggest
avenues for your own research:

(Herbs in **Bold Type** are considered particularly powerful and noteworthy. Again, the cancer types mentioned are
examples and not intended to suggest that the herb is limited
to any particular cancer.)

- Astragalus (Huang Qi). Reportedly doubles sur-
  vival times when taken with radiation therapy
- **Berberis Family** (e.g. *Podophyllum peltanum*)
  Ovarian cancer
- **Bloodroot** (*Sanguinaria canadensis*). Sarcomas
- Butcher's Broom (*Ruscus aculeatus*). Breast cancer
- **Cat's Claw** (*Uncaria tormentosa*). Skin cancers
- **Chaparral** (*Larrea mexicana*). Breast cancer
- **Curcumin** (Turmeric). All types, notably colon
  cancer.
- Dang Shen Root (*Codonopsis pilosula*). Useful for
  increasing red and white blood cell levels

- Echinacea. Brain tumors
- **Feverfew**. Leukemia
- Goldenseal. Stomach cancer
- Milk Thistle. Protects liver during chemotherapy
- Pau D'Arco. Blood and lymph
- Red Clover. Breast, prostate
- Sheep's Sorrell. General cleanser
- Skullcap (*Scutellaria barbata*). Lung, stomach
- Sutherlandia (Cancer Bush). Immune system booster
- **Thorawax** (Hare's Ear) (*Bulpleurum scorzonerae-folium*). Bone cancer
- Wheatgrass (Cleansing, anti-oxidant)
- **Wormwood** (Ching Hao, Qing Hao, Artemisinin) (*Herba Artemisiae Annuae*) General cancers, esp. leukemia)

Of all these, Wormwood (Artemisinin) strikes me as the most interesting. Artemisinin, a Chinese herb, has been used for years as a treatment for malaria. Relatively recently it has been found to be effective against cancer as well. It's been noted that cancer cells can contain up to 1,000 times the amount of iron as normal cells. Artemisinin acts against the iron, thus killing the cancer cells. There is much evidence of its anti-cancer abilities, some going so far as to call it a "cure." They may be right!

10. Can Paw Paw Be Used in Treating Animals?

Veterinary applications

Veterinary use of paw paw, one would think, would be widespread, especially among holistic vets. Not true. I researched this for weeks, sending out inquiries to veterinary colleges and veterinary associations, friends who are veterinarians, and friends of friends. "Do you ever use, or possibly know a colleague who uses paw paw to treat cancer in pet animals?" Having written two previous books dealing with pet animals, I'm pretty familiar with this territory and have several acquaintances in the veterinary profession.

Still I could come up with only single veterinarian who had any experience with paw paw and returned my inquiry. This is especially odd since veterinarians are not under the same Federal Drug Administration restrictions as "people" doctors. They are free to try "unapproved" drugs so long as the caretaker of the pet has been notified of the risks and agrees to the treatment. It's well known that new drugs are typically tested in animals before human trials are performed.

Paw paw itself was tested on dogs and found to be very well tolerated, even when given very large doses (See page 90).

I happen to have a friend who had a dog I'll call "Chelsea" that was diagnosed with bladder cancer in April of 2013.

The vets told my friend that it was inoperable, due to the tumor's location. They told him that the dog had maybe three months to live. When I learned about the case it was in May, one month later. Based on my wife's excellent progress with paw paw I suggested that he check with his veterinarians and see if they knew anything about paw paw. They apparently hadn't heard of it, but were quite willing to try it.

They gave Chelsea one capsule per day. She maintained her health until March of 2014, nearly one year after being diagnosed. The tumor did not grow during this time. She had been doing fine, no sign of cancer symptoms, lively and energetic. And suddenly, overnight, she died inexplicably. Was it the cancer that took her—or something else? That will remain unknown. But the gist of the story is that paw paw had a remarkable effect, given the dog's original diagnosis, and my friend and his family had Chelsea around for a much longer time that they had originally expected.

But, as I say, not many veterinarians are familiar with paw paw. If you have a dog or cat with cancer, you'll most likely be on your own with it, albeit it necessary to inform your vets.

Dosage suggestions

To my knowledge there is no standard dosage for pet animals. But I would venture to suggest that the guidelines for child dosage might be a starting point. That is, base the dosage upon the relative weight of the animal to a full grown human. The rule-of-thumb for a human (of, say, 200 pounds) is six capsules per day. A one-hundred-pound human, then, would take 3 capsules per day.

A fifty-pound dog, then, would take 1½ capsules per day, and so on. This would be a starting point. Round off the math to the next-highest half-capsule; I wouldn't bother with thirds and quarters. If the animal was not vomiting, one might then, ever-so-gradually, increase the dosage, ultimately to reach the maximum the animal could tolerate without vomiting. This is all undiscovered territory, since, to my knowledge, there simply are no standard guidelines for veterinary dosages—but I do think it's logical. I would suggest that whatever the total daily dosage is you don't give it all at once, one time per day. It's always better to divide the daily dose into three equal doses given at equal intervals throughout the day. Recall that capsules can be opened and their contents mixed in with food. You might try mixing the paw paw powder into a bit of raw meat or canned pet food. It's very important that it be taken with food in order to prevent vomiting.

In addition . . .

I might add that another supplement that goes well with paw paw is noni juice (See Page 72). I note that our "miracle dog" Sparky had a few tablespoons of noni every day mixed into his food. Eventually he would drink it straight! Also check out Artemisinin (see Page 76), which has been used successfully on dogs and cats with cancer. As an animal lover and pet advocate, I wish you the best of luck if your dog or your cat gets cancer. Don't give up! It *can* be beaten. Check out my website at

www.SparkyFightsBack.com

for help in finding a good oncologist and helpful natural remedies!

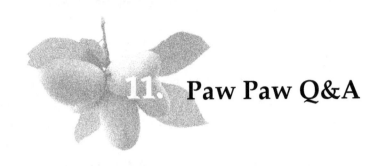

11. Paw Paw Q&A

Here's a list of answers to most questions you might have about paw paw. Many of these are related to topics I've been asked about in the past, and others are questions I had myself when first learning about the ins and outs of paw paw and related topics. The questions and their answers which follow can serve as a handy "quick reference" for any cancer patient taking paw paw.

Dr. McLaughlin's answers

Dr. Jerry McLaughlin, the chief developer and researcher of paw paw, is featured in a series of individual online videos, each clip answering a "frequently asked question" about paw paw. The following are based upon transcripts (occasionally slightly edited for clarity) of Dr. McLaughlin's live responses.[46] To view the complete videos (which I highly recommend!), go to
http://www/pawpawresearch.com/videos.html

Q. Is paw paw safe to use with traditional cancer treatments, including chemotherapy and radiation?

A. In the tests that we've conducted so far, we've had a whole various range of different types of tumors that we've had people try with paw paw, and these people had various stages, from Stage I to Stage IV. Initially, the people we had as subjects were all Stage IV. We were testing in Nevada, and the State of Nevada has a law that you can try anything if the physician and the patient agree that the patient has terminal cancer. Most of these people had already been through chemotherapy and had exhausted its potential and had gone through radiation and were, essentially, with both feet in the grave. And so we gave them paw paw.

I remember Dr. Jim Forsyth at the Reno Cancer Screening and Treatment Center, the doctor that was helping us back in 2002-2003. Jim gave us 20 cancer patients. Right away we lost seven—because they were just too far gone—but over a period of six months to a year we saw a remarkable stabilization of the health of thirteen of those patients. So, I think we can say that paw paw is safe to use. Also, Dr. Forsyth checked the usual parameters in the bloodstream for liver enzymes and for bone marrow depression and things like the white cell count, and the red cell count, and platelets and all that—the usual things that you'd want to check and make sure you're not affecting something adversely—and paw paw doesn't affect any of those at all. It worked out very well, and he was quite pleased with that. . . .

No problems with radiation either. One of our initial patients was actually one of the secretaries at the company. First she took paw paw and then she took chemo. She took five rounds of chemo and they couldn't detect the tumors anymore. And then she underwent surgery. And then she underwent radiation, and all the time she kept taking paw paw. One of the last times I saw her she had a sign on her desk that said "I'm Cancer Free."

Q. **How does paw paw work with chemotherapy to fight drug-resistant cells?**

A. We've had quite a number of people concerned about the mode of action of paw paw and how it can work in order to facilitate chemotherapy or help to maintain the effectiveness of chemotherapy. And actually, it's quite simple. Chemotherapy will run its course and after a while it doesn't work anymore — the patient becomes refractory to the effects of the chemo. The cancer becomes resistant — clinically this is called "multiple drug resistance," because a number of anti-cancer agents will not work any longer. What's happened is that the cancer cells have all developed a little pump in the cell membrane, and this little pump will pump the drug out of the cell before the drug can stay in the cell and kill the cancer cell, so the cell survives. And it doesn't make any difference what kind of chemotherapy you take, switching to another drug doesn't work, because the pump is *multiple* drug resistant, and it pumps all compounds out. . . .

Furthermore, [paw paw acetogenins] inhibit the pump mechanism. The pump requires energy, and the energy comes in the form of adenosine tri-phosphate, or "ATP." So by inhibiting ATP production, which is the mode of action of the paw paw material — in the mitochondria as well as in the cell membrane and ADH oxidation system — we end up decreasing the ATP concentration so that the pump won't work. And so there isn't any energy to run the pump.

So if we would give paw paw *with* chemo at that stage we would allow the chemo to stay in the cell longer. And maybe we can *restore* the effectiveness of the chemotherapy by giving paw paw with the chemo in refractory patients. Furthermore, if we would give the paw paw earlier on with the chemo, we would prevent a resistance from developing, because the paw paw would help to kill off the resistant cells as they develop. So it makes sense to me to give paw paw with chemo to prevent further resistance from developing. Paw paw alone will work, but the two together will work [synergistically].

Q. **Can the use of paw paw reduce the need for higher chemotherapy dosage over time?**

A. I would say that, in patients who have repeat cancer (they've been through remission, and now the cancer's coming back), quite often they have to have more and more chemo, diverse types of chemo, and higher doses of the chemo, so that eventually you get to the point where the side effects of the chemo become so debilitating that the patient would rather die, and it doesn't work any longer.

Paw paw can help to prevent that from happening, because paw paw kills resistant cells. It kills resistant cells better. Even in the *cockroach* study that we did we were able to kill pesticide resistant cockroaches with some of the paw paw compounds at one fifth the concentration that it took to kill the normal cockroaches that didn't have any resistance! So the same is true of cancer cells. And the pesticide resistance, incidentally, is an ATP dependent process as well. Just like cancer cell resistance, multiple drug resistance in cancer is ATP dependent.

So it makes sense to give paw paw in these cases, and let's keep those doses down, and we can help patients by helping to alleviate some of those devastating side effects of the chemo and keep them alive longer—which is what it's all about—with quality of life, without being sick.

Q. **What did Upjohn Co. (now Pfizer) find when they ran tests comparing paw paw to the chemotherapy drug Taxol?**

A. We've done a head-to-head comparison of Taxol with paw paw. This was done not by me but what was then the Upjohn company—it's now Pfizer—and they tested it against L1210 leukemia—mouse (murine) leukemia. [Here's how these tests are conducted.] You look at the number of days the mice will live. Usually the mice will live for ten days with leukemia; then the leukemia will kill them. If the mice can live for twelve days or longer then it's considered to be significant. With Taxol and with paw paw we had the mice living in the range of fourteen days or so. So that was "active."

But— the Taxol mice lost 10% of their bodyweight in that ten-day period, showing that they were extremely poisoned by Taxol. And we know that Taxol is a cardio-toxic material and also is neuro-toxic (tingling in the fingers and all that)—so that Taxol is nasty. But, with the paw paw compound, we had a 5% *increase* in bodyweight in that time—they didn't lose weight. They were happy; they weren't *sick*. And this is from actually *injecting* the paw paw material, as well. So, it is possible to inject paw paw, but it doesn't make sense to me to inject anything when you can take it orally. And, by taking it orally, if you happen to give too much, vomiting is your safety valve and you can throw it up. If you inject it you can't get it back; it's in there. And if it's too much for a particular individual it would be curtains then. So I feel very safe with paw paw as an orally-administered [material].

Q. Can a person start out with a lower dosage to test its effect?

A. With a number of cancer patients who are already on chemo or who are a little bit apprehensive about trying paw paw in the first place—who worry about allergies or whatever—it makes sense to try one paw paw the first day, one capsule. The second day two, third day three, fourth day four. Then you're off and running with four, which is the usual amount. That makes sense to me. If you're taking chemo, and you're already [queasy] on the chemo—because chemo causes nausea and vomiting—there's a possibility that there might be added nausea and vomiting induced by paw paw. I haven't really seen it, but there's a possibility. So in that case, again, start with a small, tolerable dose of the paw paw, and work your way up. Heavier people get up to taking eight, and even twelve paw paw capsules.

Q. Can paw paw be used with radiation therapy?

A. The question is easy to answer. The answer is "yes." We've had no problems whatsoever with people taking radiation concurrently with paw paw or either before or after paw paw. Paw paw doesn't seem to affect any of the mechanisms that you'd understand for ionizing radiation, so it seems like [it's] no problem.

Q. Is paw paw safe to use with other alternative cancer treatments, including antioxidants?

A. Initially, with antioxidants, according to the mechanism of action of paw paw, high doses of antioxidants would interfere with the mode of action of paw paw and help to prevent program cell death (which is what we want to have happen with paw paw). And antioxidants help prevent program cell death because they involve, probably, hydrogen peroxide. And that would destroy the hydrogen peroxide. So initially I said we shouldn't be giving paw paw with antioxidants.

Well, now I understand that after Bill Keller and Fred Valeriote. (Fred is at Wayne State University) have done a study. And Fred has a very interesting little biological assay that he uses with Petri dishes and lines of cancer cells that are growing in culture. And you can put a disk in there of anticancer material and you'll get a zone of inhibition, just like with antibiotic testing with bacteria or fungi. He did that test and found that if you put antioxidants and paw paw together he actually got a better effect and not a lesser effect. So I would say that I was wrong, that we can use antioxidants with paw paw as alternative treatment.

Actually, with enzymes, like high levels of proteases, we initially came out and recommended that these be taken with paw paw. And with immuno-stimulants, some of the polysaccharides, the beta glucans—these products definitely can be taken with the paw paw.

So I don't know of any interfering effects of alternative treatments. Some people with essiac tea, and burdock root (which is one of the components of essiac tea)—I've heard that they've taken both with paw paw and there's been no problems with the effects.

Of course there's the "PC–SPES" stuff, which was for prostate cancer "hope"—which was a farce, because it actually contains diethylstilbestrol.[47] And it was causing clotting problems because estrogens cause clotting problems. So then they laced it with warfarin, an anticoagulant, and that was not a good idea. The federal government tested it and found out those problems, and from that all natural materials got a bad name as being fake and toxic.

With paw paw I think I can safely say that there are very few natural anticancer remedies or alleviants or adjuvants that have had as much research as paw paw.

Q. With what kinds of cancer has paw paw been used successfully?

A. We had seen since we tested with ninety-some cancer patients these people had a broad range of cancers. Actually, we didn't have very many leukemia patients; we had some childhood leukemia patients, but I don't have any real conclusions that I can draw from that.

Lymphomas, another type of soft cancer, definitely we had good effects there—and actually one lady in Australia I feel we kept going for quite some time. She did pass away, but we're not sure if it was from the complications of some of the previous chemotherapy she'd had.

Melanomas—we've had one really dramatic case of melanoma with a patient in Oklahoma, but on the other hand I've had one disappointing case where a close friend of mine had melanoma and, in spite of paw paw, passed away. His wife told me that she's not quite sure if he was really taking the paw paw as he was supposed to. So I'm not really sure it was a good test case.

All of the cases that I can relate are people who were essentially volunteers to take this, and if they choose not take it and don't tell anybody, you don't really know. It's not really a clinical study where someone's forcing them to take the medicine, forcing them to take the supplement.

Q. **Can paw paw be used topically for skin cancers such as melanoma?**

A. I'd have to say I don't know. I have put the paw paw into an ointment base with golden salve, and it is actually quite remarkable for the different things that it will do. It's really good against fungi, such as athlete's foot, and some folks have had relief from eczema and dermatitis of different types, and all that. But I'm not sure— I've also put it on insect bites, such as bee stings, and it seems to help.

But whether or not it's going to help with melanoma, I don't really know. Theoretically it should. It could help to dry up the skin lesions, but if someone has melanoma, *surgery* is definitely the first thing they should do—and get it cut out with as wide an area as tolerable of surrounding tissue. And then you have to look for lumps forming in the regional lymph nodes, such as the sub-axillary—under the arm lymph nodes—and hope that it doesn't happen. If it happens, and it's malignant melanoma, the patient usually has less than a year.

Q. **Are there any known problems with using paw paw with any known medications?**

A. I'd have to say we don't know of any problems. Quite often, if someone's going in for surgery, since they don't want any anticoagulant effects—some coumarins or anything in the natural material— they recommend discontinuing the herbal material two weeks before the surgery. That's just a rule-of-thumb that I know the company uses and the health science people there advise people to do that. That covers them—whether it's real or not as to the necessity, I don't believe so. I would suggest that you continue to take paw paw right along with other medications prior to surgery and all that. It certainly doesn't have an anticoagulant effect.

Q. **Can paw paw be used as a cancer preventative?**

A. "Can paw paw be used as a cancer preventative?"—I get this question all the time. People would like to take paw paw preventatively, especially because it's not very expensive. My answer to that is "Would you take an antibiotic every day to keep yourself from getting an infection?" And the answer is "no"—you wait until you get an infection and then you take the antibiotic of choice.

I think with paw paw this is what you should do: If you have a cancer, then definitely you should take it. There are cases where we've had, say, ladies with breast cancer who had, say, lumpectomies and then followed with chemo and surgery taking paw paw all the time and then taking paw paw for six months or so afterwards, and then alternating months—take paw paw one month; don't take it the next month, [etc.]. It's really not a study that I'm talking about [but] a few cases where this procedure has been followed and the cancers have not come back.

So, I think that in that case there's a good reason to be taking it as a cancer preventative because you've already had cancer. If cancer is in the family and it's likely that you are going to get it, perhaps it would be wise to take it preventatively.

Q. **What is the optimum dosage? Can you take more or less? How should you space the dosages each day?**

A. Well, as a supplement, you're supposed to say "serving size" instead of "dosage," but the initial cancer patients who took paw paw took the equivalent of two capsules at a time, four times a day—so that means like eight capsules a day. And these were three ladies, all with terminal ovarian cancer—and they all three vomited. So—we gave them too much. After that we decided to try half that amount—and they didn't vomit.

I'd worked out the initial quantity to take based on dogs—because that's what we had to go on, beagle dogs. And, with the beagles, we got up to 32 capsules at a time four times a day—and we couldn't kill the dogs; they just vomited. So I think you can probably take the paw paw up until the amount that causes you to be nauseated and vomiting. I know there are a lot of people right now that are taking six and eight a day instead of four a day, especially if the people are heavier, say 200 pounds or more. If someone's 99 pounds, then probably four a day is enough, and maybe even three a day might do it.

But for children, I have just sort of based things proportionately on their weight. If it's a child that weighs 50 pounds with leukemia, for example, we just take a quarter of the amount. Say an average adult would be about 170-200 pounds, 50 pounds would be roughly one fourth of that, so give them the equivalent of one capsule per day. You can pull the capsules apart, divide the pile of powder into four little piles, put it into some apple sauce and kids take it.

How should you space the dosages? Well, back in "Pharmacokinetics 101"—in pharmacy school you'll learn about blood levels of materials. And if you take an injection of something, for example, the blood level goes right up. But then it falls off. And there has to be a certain blood level which is the minimum for the material to be effective. So, if we give an oral dose of the material, say the minimum effective level is [at a certain point] and we go up above [to a higher point], and we don't want it to drop the blood level down below [the minimum level], we want to give another dose before we get down to that level. We want to keep it up there; we don't want it going down and then coming back up. So that means spacing things out as evenly as possible.

So every six hours would be four times a day. Now, the practical side of this is usually breakfast, lunch, dinner, and bedtime. And with paw paw, it's best if you take it with something (drink some milk; eat some food; take it with a meal). A lot of people slip a couple capsules in their shirt pocket, and if they're away from home and they don't have the bottle they can just reach and grab a capsule and take it with the MacDonald's hamburger or whatever they're eating.

Q. **What is the benefit of using Mangosteen juice or other strong antioxidants with paw paw?**

A. That goes back to the use of antioxidants with paw paw, and as I mentioned before, Dr. Keller and Dr. Valeriote have performed combination studies *in vitro* (in glass and Petri dishes) demonstrating that paw paw with antioxidants actually has an additive effect or maybe even a synergistic effect—and certainly is not inhibitive. So I would say take it with those antioxidants. The mangosteen, as I recall, we were developing that at the company just as I was leaving. Part of the rationale for using that mangosteen product was that we tested all kinds of juices and materials in this HORAC[48] test—and the HORAC test showed that the mangosteen was one of the highest of the natural materials in the HORAC value.

Q. **What are the differences between paw paw and graviola?**

A. Graviola is another species of fruit tree in the *Annonaceae* family. The Spanish name for it is *guanábana* (maybe some of you would recognize it by that name). The French name is *corassol*; the English name is soursop; the Dutch name is *zuurzak*—and the Brazilian name, the Portuguese name, is graviola.

There are at least a couple products that are just the powdered leaves of graviola, and twigs. . . . The scientific name of graviola is *Annona muricata,* and if you look in the literature I have identified, I'd say, I think at least 28 compounds from *Annona muricata.*

We had a big project on the seeds and another big project on the leaves. Both of them contained acetogenic compounds, but the graviola product only contained a single ring of acetogenic compounds. Paw paw is so powerful because it has the double ring compounds. And we performed structure activity relationships for many, many compounds—with well over 50 compounds in this *Annonaceae* class of acetogenins. The single ring compounds are *many* times less potent than the double ring compounds. And so graviola doesn't contain the most powerful compounds.

We did some tests at the company, and demonstrated that the other products that are out there are 20 to 50 times less potent than the paw paw product in capsule form. We did that test. It's a very simple test, using brine shrimp.[49] . . . You can test biological materials that way. Actually, that's how we standardize paw paw. To start, we standardize it with the brine shrimp test to make sure that all the lots are similar and their potency is consistent from capsule to capsule, bottle to bottle. You don't run into that consistency or that biological standardization with these competing products.

Their scientists do not standardize the stuff; they just assume that the leaves are potent. They may be collected at the wrong time of year. I'll tell you, if you collect paw paw leaves in the fall, they're worthless. There are some flavonoids in there, but actually they start to decompose with fungi and stuff attacking them. So, the time of collection is extremely important. We've worked this all out with paw paw—this is stuff that I did basically, to know that basically in the month of May is when you want to collect the paw paw twigs. And the twigs are the most logical source of renewable biomass, so that we don't have to kill the trees by stripping the bark from trees. . . . These tests have not been done with graviola—these seasonal variations tests, [which] part of the plant [to use] and all that haven't been really standardized.

—o—

I trust that by now you have a more complete picture of just what paw paw is, and what it does. Now I'd like to move on from the scientific aspects of paw paw, and get a bit motivational. . . .

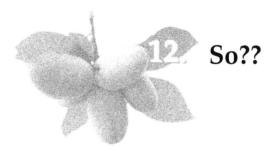

So??

I direct this final message straight to the cancer patient. You are the reason I have written this book. In the final analysis you will be the one to make all decisions regarding what treatments you will accept and what you will reject. I have some personal appreciation of the position you are now in. I imagine that practically everyone at some time in their life has been touched, directly or indirectly, by this challenging, most unfortunate disease.

My immediate family at home has consisted simply of my wife, myself, and our dog. All three of us have been cancer patients. Josée, long before her recent cancer episodes (simultaneous lung and uterine cancers), first came down with lung cancer in 1983. Fortunately it was a single, resectable tumor—but I remember the fear, the trauma of going through that experience, culminating with surgery, which left her with only one lobe remaining in her left lung. And the healing process was agonizing. The operation involved breaking several ribs. She was in pain for several months until all was healed.

I also recall, in the year 2000, the shock of being told that our terrier Sparky had lymphoma, and that his chances of surviving for more than a year were not very good. What an emotion-filled, roller coaster year that was—before his final triumph! We still think of it as a miracle.

A few years earlier, in 1998, my urologist suspected something going on in my prostate. He took a biopsy and I awaited the results, which he would relay by phone. I was teaching high school at the time. One of my functions was pi-ano accompanist for school functions and concerts. The an-nual school musical, *A Chorus Line* that year, was in rehearsal, and I was the pianist—providing the sole musical accompa-niment for the show. Just before the curtain rose on the open-ing night performance I received the call: It was cancer. What an effort it took to play that show—fighting off the myriad thoughts exploding in my brain while my fingers rattled over the keys! "Kiss today good-bye, and point me to tomorrow" indeed! [50]

Subsequently, after considering all the options, I had ra-dioactive seeds implanted, and the results were good. I still must go in for checkups every six months. Once you've been a cancer patient, even if ostensibly cured, you must be ob-served and checked for the rest of your life. And presently, even after Josée's remission, we must remain ever vigilant. Fighting cancer never really "ends."

Making decisions about treatments for cancer are never easy. I have tried, within these pages, to make a case for what I consider to be a most promising option. If you've read this far, I hope that I have opened your mind to a course you oth-erwise may not have taken. But I'm aware how resistant some people can be to trying something new or out of the ordinary. I have a neighbor who has been fighting metastatic bladder cancer for some time. After my wife had had such good pro-gress with paw paw, I told this lady about it. I typed up all the references I had—where she could go online to learn more—all the information I thought would be helpful, and gave it to her. She never responded one way or the other, and the next time I ran into her she didn't even mention anything about it.

I have a longtime friend, a senior, who I learned had lung cancer. I informed him of Josée's success, etc., and recommended paw paw and gave him all the information. He indicated that he would definitely look into it. But again, that was it. Nothing further was said.

There must be many people with the inclination to trust only in standard treatments. Their doctors know best, and if their doctor doesn't know about it how can there possibly be any value to it? I agree that doctors can be great. They take their work very seriously. The vast majority are sympathetic and understanding, competent, and know what they are doing.

But they don't know *everything*. No one does. Standard medicine, as it stands today, is quite limited in what it can provide in terms of treating and, most importantly, *curing* cancer.

Roughly one out of every three people (32%) on standard treatment today for some type of cancer will not live longer than five years. Suppose I held up three cards and told you to pick a card without looking. One of the cards, I would explain, is the Ace of Spades. The other two are random. If you picked one of the random cards you would be cured. If you picked the Ace of Spades you would be dead within five years. Would you do it? That's the bet you are making on today's standard cancer treatments!

True, there are many very promising new treatments now in development, from gene therapy to immunotherapy to virotherapy to many other novel techniques. Eventually,

perhaps sooner rather than later, the current "big three" —
chemotherapy, radiation, and surgery — will become obsolete.
Meanwhile, however, they remain dominant. [51] And, believe
me, they will die a hard death. What would standard medicine do without them, and the income they produce by *not*
swiftly curing so many cancer patients?

Figures for 2010 showed that the total cost of treating
cancer in the United States was 125 billion dollars. By 2020
this figure is projected to be 158 billion.[52] A single 8-week
cycle of chemotherapy can run as much as $30,000.[53]

The scale is huge when it comes to the cancer industry.
Yes, *industry* — it's big business, with three overwhelming
components:

First, the Medical Industry. Don't get me wrong; as I've
said, there are many, *many* medical professionals — doctors,
nurses, technicians, assistants, advisors, *et al* — who are caring,
sincere, dedicated people who truly have the patient's needs
at heart. But the *industry* is in the business of making money.
And cancer is a big part of that to say the least. Where in this
is the motivation to cure cancer? Imagine that tomorrow that
magic bullet was discovered. The bottom would fall out. Facilities would have to close their doors while people scramble
to keep their jobs.

Second, there's Big Pharma. It takes millions of dollars to
develop a new patentable cancer drug, more millions to test it
and get it approved by the FDA, then more to advertise it and
market it. Where would they be if suddenly someone came up
with a drug that could cure cancer in a matter of days? Is it
any wonder that while a cure has been sought for over a hun-
dred years Big Pharma has not yet come up with one?

And the third player—Government. Why, oh why aren't they funding clinical trials for non-patentable promising natural remedies? They can pass out grants for studies of the mating habits of barn owls or whatever, but for natural cancer treatments—? Remember that natural substances, in and of themselves, can't be patented. You can't patent extract from the bark of a yew tree, but you can synthesize it, call

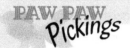

Cost of Researching a New Drug

For every new drug that is approved, the average spent on research and development is $4 billion.
- Matthew Herper, in *Forbes*

it Paclitaxel and make millions on it. But some natural drugs are just too (often beneficially) complicated to synthesize. No patent. No millions. And so no clinical trials. Where better could the government spend our hard-earned money than on this? But they don't. Makes you wonder just how much Big Pharma money is ending up in the pockets of elected government officials and bureaucrats.

And that's the State of the Industry.

So along comes this book about an extract that comes from the twigs of a tree and costs less than $50 a month (along with survival rate statistics that might put chemo to shame!). I believe the research has been extensive and convincing. The track record and the case histories are exceptionally promising. But I realize that some will consider paw paw just more quackery based on false promises designed only to lighten their wallet. They've just "never heard of it before" (and neither has their oncologist), and so mistrust it. And, quite likely, they are wary of a layman such as myself. And I understand that—I make no claim to being a medical expert; I'm simply an investigative reporter, relaying the product of my research. I might point out, however, that as an independent individual I have no professional axe to grind, and no professional colleagues to support or defend. I do understand, though, how unfamiliar ideas can be held suspect.

But—*what's the big deal?* What great *risk* are you taking if you decide to try paw paw?

Are you going to spend a fortune? Certainly not. Paw paw is, even compared to other natural/alternative treatments, practically the least expensive natural anticancer supplement you can buy! In New York State, where I live, you would pay more for four packs of cigarettes than a month's supply of paw paw (irony intended).[54]

Are you concerned about side effects? We've shown here that there are virtually no serious side effects if taken correctly as advised. In all the clinical studies, not a single serious side effect was reported. It's amazing that anyone who has chosen to accept the normal—often debilitating—side effects of chemotherapy and/or radiation would be concerned about the side effects of paw paw!

So now, as I close, I have but one wish—that you will at least *try* paw paw, alone or in concert with standard treatments. I venture to say that you have nothing to lose. Paw paw, as noted earlier, will not negatively affect other treatments you are undergoing, such as chemo or radiation therapies. In fact, it stands to *increase* their effectiveness. And, when you try it, remember that paw paw works slowly. Don't expect overnight success. Give it time before making an evaluation of your progress, say, 3-6 months. And remember that *no* treatment works on absolutely *everybody*.

Check with your oncologist; inform him/her of what you are doing. If they seem curious, give them a copy of this book—why not?

Do further research if you like. You will find more information online (check *References* at the end of this book), and there is a least one other book on the topic.[55] Remember that you are not alone. Thousands of others have successfully used paw paw. You are *not* experimenting or grasping at straws!

If you are unaccustomed to thinking "outside the box," I urge you to make a significant exception. That is the hope that goes out with every copy of this book, along with a prayer for your well-being and your success.

Notes

[1] See *Sparky Fights Back,* Josée Clerens and John Clifton, Foley Square Books, 2005

[2] Jerome Groopman, M.D., *The Anatomy of Hope,* 2004

[3] American Cancer Society, *Carboplatin,* *http://www.cancer.org/treatment/treatmentsandsideeffects/guidetocancerdrugs/carboplatin*

[4] American Cancer society, *Paclitaxel,* *http://www.cancer.org/treatment/treatmentsandsideeffects/guidetocancerdrugs/paclitaxel*

[5] American Cancer Society, *Filgrastim* (commercial name Neupogen), *http://www.cancer.org/treatment/treatmentsandsideeffects/guidetocancerdrugs/filgrastim*

[6] American Cancer Society, *Pemetrexed* (commercial name Alimta), *http://www.cancer.org/treatment/treatmentsandsideeffects/guidetocancerdrugs/pemetrexed*

[7] Mayo Clinic, *Positron Emission Tomography (PET) scan,* *http://www.mayoclinic.org/tests-procedures/pet-scan/basics/definition/prc-20014301*

[8] The Common paw paw *(Asimina triloba)* is a species of paw paw, native to eastern North America, from southernmost Ontario and New York west to eastern Nebraska, and south to northern Florida and eastern Texas. —Wikipedia.org

[9] *Buying Louisiana: An Eyewitness's Account of the Louisiana Purchase.* Josée Clerens, New ed. 2014

[10] Memorial Sloane Kettering—Cancer Center, *Graviola.* http://www.mskcc.org/cancer-care/herb/graviola

[11] Paw Paw Research, *Graviola.* http://www.pawpawresearch.com/graviola-inferior.html

[12] Feras Q. Alali, Xiao-Xi Liu, and Jerry L. McLaughlin, Department of Medicinal Chemistry and Molecular Pharmacology, School of Pharmacy and Pharmacal Sciences, *Annonaceous Acetogenins: Recent Progress,* Purdue University, September 18, 1998 , *http://alternativecancer.us/acetogenins1999.pdf*

[13] Chemotherapy drugs also seek out the fastest growing cells. However, chemotherapy is designed to poison the cells as opposed to depriving them of energy, as does paw paw.

[14] Navdeep S. Chandel, *Mitochondria and cancer, 2014, http://www.cancerandmetabolism.com/content/2/1/8*

[15] *How Paw Paw Works Against Cancer Cells, http://pawpawresearch.com/pawpawworks.html*

[16] *http://dictionary.sensagent.com*, Pharmacognosy (n.) The science of drugs prepared from natural sources including preparations from plants, animals, and other organisms as well as minerals and other substances included in *materia medica*.

[17] McLaughlin's associates have included Gina B. Benson, Ching-jer Chang, Vicki L. Croy, James Forsythe M.D., Marietta L. Harrison, and Nicholas H. Oberlies, among others.

[18] Graeme Morgan, Robyn Ward, Michael Barton, *The Contribution of Cytotoxic Chemotherapy to 5-year Survival in Adult Malignancies*, 2004, *https://www.burtongoldberg.com/home/burtongoldberg/contribution-of-chemotherapy-to-five-year-survival-rate-morgan.pdf*

[19] Janet Raloff, *Look what's Hidden in the Pawpaw Tree Fruit*, Science News, Feb. 29, 1992 (*http://pawpawresearch.com/hidden-article.html*)

[20] Ibid.

[21] Ibid.

[22] Purdue News, 1997, *Paw Paw Shows Promise in Fighting Drug-Resistant Tumors*, reprinted in *http://pawpawresearch.com/purdue-mdr-97.html*

[23] These mechanisms are called "P-glycoprotein mediated pumps."

[24] *A novel mechanism for the control of clinical cancer. Inhibition of the productions of adenosine triphosphate (ATP) with a standardized extract off paw paw (asimina triloba, Annonaceae)*, Jerry L. McLaughlin Ph D., Gina B. Benson, and James Forsythe M.D. *http://pawpawresearch.com/pawpaw-trials1.pdf*

[25] "Prostate Specific Antigen" (PSA) tests measure the presence of cancerous activity in the prostate gland.

[26] Lorene Benoit, *The Paw Paw Program: A "Christopher Columbus" Approach to Cancer*, (Duncan, BC, Canada: Benoit and Associates Health, 2010) 120-162

[27] Brian D. Lawenda, M.D., *Is There Any Other Anti-Cancer Botanical Compound As Exciting As Curcumin?* March 18, 2013. *http://www.integrativeoncology-essentials.com/2013/03/is-there-any-other-anti-cancer-botanical-compound-as-exciting-as-curcumin/#sthash.SSBRmr9X.dpuf*

[28] Jerry L. McLaughlin Ph D., Gina B. Benson, and James Forsythe M.D. *A novel mechanism for the control of clinical cancer. Inhibition of the productions of adenosine triphosphate (ATP) with a standardized extract off paw paw (asimina triloba, Annonaceae)*, page 1, *http://pawpawresearch.com/pawpaw-trials1.pdf*

[29] See 19

[30] Graeme Morgan, Robyn Ward, Michael Barton, *The Contribution of Cytotoxic Chemotherapy to 5-year Survival in Adult Malignancies*, 2004 *https://www.burtongoldberg.com/home/burtongoldberg/contribution-of-chemotherapy-to-five-year-survival-rate-morgan.pdf*

[31] See 19

[32] National Cancer Institute, *Radiation Therapy for Cancer*, *http://www.cancer.gov/cancertopics/factsheet/Therapy/radiation*

[33] American Cancer Society, *How is surgery used for cancer?*, *http://www.cancer.org/treatment/treatmentsandsideeffects/treatmenttypes/surgery/surgery-how-is-surgery-used-for-cancer*

[34] Michael Stanclift, N.D., *You're What Kind of Doctor?*, *http://www.huffingtonpost.com/michael-stanclift-nd/naturopathic-doctors_b_1923371.html*

[35] *http://www.naturopathic.org/AF_MemberDirectory.asp?version=2*

[36] The Pawpaw/Asimina triloba/Scientific Paper, *http://pawpaws.net/Pawpaw_Scientific_Paper.htm*

[37] Dr. Jerry McLaughlin. *Can paw paw be used as a cancer preventative?*, *http://pawpawresearch.com/videos.html*

[38] catabolism: n. The metabolic breakdown of complex molecules into simpler ones, often resulting in a release of energy.

[39] Lorene Benoit, *The Paw Paw Program: A "Christopher Columbus" Approach to Cancer*,(Duncan, BC, Canada: Benoit and Associates Health, 2010) 257

[40] How Antioxidants work, WebMD, *http://www.webmd.com/food-recipes/features/how-antioxidants-work1*

[41] Mangosteen, Drugs.com, *http://www.drugs.com/npp/mangosteen.html*

[42] Paw Paw Research, *Positive Results from Combining Paw Paw with Thai-Go™ Mangosteen Juice Blend*, *http://pawpawresearch.com/pawpaw-mangosteen.html*

[43] Neil Solomon MD, PhD, *The Noni Phenomenon*, November 23, 1999

[44] *www.tahitinaturel.us*

[45] See 27

[46] McLaughlin, Jerry, *Video Questions and Answers with Dr. Jerry McLaughlin*, *http://pawpawresearch.com/videos.html*

[47] Diethylstilbestrol (DES) is a synthetic form of the female hormone estrogen. *See* National Cancer Institute, *Diethylstilbestrol (DES) and Cancer*, *http://www.cancer.gov/cancertopics/factsheet/Risk/DES*

[48] HORAC test: "Hydroxyl Radical Antioxidant Capacity" assay (test) for determining antioxidant levels in a material

[49] Brine Shrimp: A Convenient General Bioassay for Active Plant Constituents, B. N. Meyer, N. R. Ferrigni*, J. E. Putnam, L. B. Jacobsen, D. E. Nichols and J. L. McLaughlin, January,1982, *http://www.researchgate.net/publication/51380045_Brine_shrimp_a_convenient_general_bioassay_for_active_plant_constituents*

[50] *What I Did for Love*, lyric by Ed Kleban, music by Marvin Hamlisch

[51] Many observers have noted that it is more lucrative for the big drug companies to produce products that treat cancer rather than ones that can cure it. This is axiomatically true in the sense that curing the disease would eliminate repeat sales. However, I have seen no evidence that drug companies are actually withholding a cure—though the possibility cannot be ruled out.

[52] National Institute of Health *http://www.nih.gov/news/health/jan2011/nci-12.htm*

[53] Ritwik Ghosh, *The Average Cost for Cancer Chemotherapy Treatment*, LiveStrong.com, August 16, 2013, *http://www.livestrong.com/article/153376-the-average-cost-for-cancer-chemotherapy-treatment/*

[54] The current average price in New York State for a pack of cigarettes (tax included) is $12.85

[55] *See* 25

[56] *john@johnclifton.net*, An extensive bibliography is provided.

[57] This book was a finalist for Best Book Award, Dog Writers of America, 2005.

References

Scientific papers

Ahammadsahib KI, Hollingworth RM, McGovren JP, Hui YH, McLaughlin JL, "Mode of action of bullatacin: a potent antitumor and pesticidal agent," *Life Sciences,* 1993, 53 (14):1113-1120.

Alali FQ, Liu XW, McLaughlin JL, "Annonaceous acetogenins: recent progress," *Journal of Natural Products,* 1999, 62 (3):504-540.

Alfonso D, Johnson HA, Colman-Saizarbitoria T. Presley CP, McCabe GP, McLaughlin JL, "SARs of annonaceous acetogenins in rat liver mitochondria," *Natural Toxins.* 1996, 4 (4):181-188 and Erratum 1996; 4 (6):295.

Avalos J, Rupprecht JK, McLaughlin JL, Rodriguez E, "Guinea pig maximization test of the bark extract of paw paw," *Contact Dermatitis,* 1993, 29 (1):33-35.

Ayre SG, Garcia y Bellon DP, Garcia Jr. DP, "Insulin, chemotherapy, and the mechanisms of malignancy: the design and the demise of cancer," *Medical Hypothesis,* 2000, 55 (4):330-334.

Chih HW, Chiu HF, Tang KS, Chang FR, Wu YC,. "Bullatacin, a potent antitumor annonaceous acetogenin, inhibits proliferation of human hepatocarcinoma cell line 2.2.15 by apoptosis induction," *Life Sciences,* 2001, 69 (11):1321-1331.

Chiu HF, Chih TT, Hsian YM, Tseng CH, Wu MJ, Wu YC, "Bullatacin, a potent antitumor annonaceous acetogenin, induces apoptosis through a reduction of intracellular cAMP and cGMP levels in human hepatoma 2.2.15 cells," *Biochemical Pharmacology,* 2003, 65 (3):319-327.

Cullen JK, Yee D, Sly WS, Purdue J, Hampton B,Lippman ME, Rosen N, "Insulin-like growth factor receptor expression and function in human breast cancer," *Cancer Research*, 1990, 50 (1):48-53.

Fang XP, Rieser MJ, Gu ZM, Zhao GX, McLaughlin JL, "Annonaceous acetogenins: an updated review," *Phytochemical Analysis*, 1993, 4 (1):27-48 (part 1) and 49-67 (part 2).

Fu LW, Pan QC, Liang YJ, Huang HB, "Circumvention of tumor multidrug resistance by a new annonaceous acetogenin: atemoyacin-B," *Zhongguo Yao Li Xue Bao*, 1999, 20 (5):435-439.

Gu ZM, Johnson HA, Zhou D, Wu J, Gordon J, McLaughlin JL, "Quantitative evaluation of annonaceous acetogenins in monthly samples of paw paw (Asimina triloba) twigs by liquid chromatography/electrospray ionization/tandem mass spectrometry," *Phytochemical Analysis*, 1999, 10 (1):32-38.

Gu ZM, Zeng L, Fang XP, Colman-Saizarbitoria T, Huo M, McLaughlin JL,. "Determining absolute configurations of stereocenters in annonaceous acetogenins through formaldehyde acetal derivatives and Mosher ester methodology," *Journal of Organic Chemistry*, 1994, 59 (18): 5162-5172.

Gu ZM, Zhao GX, Oberlies NH, Zeng L, McLaughlin JL, "Annonaceous acetogenins: mitochondrial inhibitors with diverse applications,". In: Arnason JT, Mata R, Romeo JT, eds., *Recent Advances in Phytochemistry. New York, NY: Plenum Press*, 1995, 249-310.

Gu ZM, Zhou D, Wu J, Shi G, Zeng L, McLaughlin JL, "Screening for Annonaceous acetogenins in bioactive plant extracts by liquid chromatography/mass spectrometry," *Journal of Natural Products*, 1997, 60 (3):242-248.

Guadano A, Gutierrez C, de la Pena E, Cortes D, Gonzales-Coloma A, "Insecticidal and mutagenic evaluation of two annonaceous acetogenins," *Journal of Natural Products*, 2000, 63 (6): 773-776.

Guadano A, Gutierrez C, de la Pena E, Cortes D, and Gonzales-Coloma S, "Insecticidal and mutagenic evaluation of two annonaceous acetogenins," *Journal of Natural Products*, 2000, 63 773-776.

He K, Shi G, Zhao GX, Zeng L, Ye Q, Schwedler JT, Wood KV, McLaughlin JL, "Three new adjacent bis-tetrahydrofuran acetogenins with four hydroxyl groups from Asimina trilobu," *Journal of Natural Products*, 1996, 59 (11):1029-1034.

He K, Zhao GX, Shi G, Zen- L, Chao JF, McLaughlin JL, "Additional bioactive annonaceous acetogenins from Asimina triloba (Annonaceae)," *Bioorganic and Medicinal Chemistry*, 1997, 5 (3):501-506.

He K, Zhao GX, Shi G, Zeng L, Chao JF, and McLaughlin JL, "Additional bioactive annonaceous acetogenins from Asimina triloba (Annonaceae)," *Bioorganic and Medicinal Chemistry*, 1997, 5 501-506.

Hollingworth RM, Ahammadsahib KI, Gadelhak G, McLaughlin JL, "New inhibitors of complex I of the mitochondrial electron transport chain with activity as pesticides," *Biochemical Society Transactions*, 1994, 22 (1):230-233.

Hollingworth, PM, Ahammadsahib KI, Gadelhak G, and McLaughlin JL, "New inhibitors of complex I of the mitochondrial electron transport chain with activity as pesticides," *Biochemical Society Transactions*, 1994, 22, 230-233.

Hopp DC, Zeng L, Gu ZM, Kozlowski JF, McLaughlin JL, "Novel mono-tetrahydrofuran ring acetogenins, from the bark of Annona squamosa, showing cytotoxic selectivities for the human pancreatic carcinoma cell line, PACA-2," *Journal of Natural Products*, 1997, 60 (6):581586.

Hopp DC, Zeng L, Gu ZM, McLaughlin JL, "Squamotacin: an annonaceous acetogenin with cytotoxic selectivity for the human prostate tumor cell line (PC-3)," *Journal of Natural Products*, 1996, 59 (2):97-99.

Hui YH, Rupprecht JK, Anderson JE, Liu YM, Smith DL, Chang CJ, McLaughlin JL. "Bullatalicin, a novel bioactive acetogenin from Annona bullata(Annonaceae)," *Tetrahedron*, 1989 45 (22):6941-6948.

Hui YH, Rupprecht JK, Liu YM, Anderson JE, Smith DL, Chang CJ, McLauahlin JL, "Bullatacin and bullatacinone: two highly potent bioactive acetogenins from Annona bullata," *Journal of Natural Products*, 1989, 52 (3):463-477.

Hui YH, Rupprecht JK, Anderson JE, Liu YM, Smith DL, Chang CJ, and McLaughlin JL, "Bullatalicin, a novel bioactive acetogenin from Annona bullata (Annonaceae)," *Tetrahedron*, 1989, 45 6941-6948.

Hui YH, Rupprecht JK, Liu YM, Anderson JE, Smith DL, Chang, CJ and McLaughlin JL, "Bullatacin and bullatacinone: two highly potent bioactive acetogenins from Annona bullta," *Journal of Natural Products*, 1989, 52 463-477.

Johnson HA, Oberlies NH, Alali FQ, McLaughlin JL, "Thwarting resistance: annonaceous acetogenins as new pesticidal and antitumor agents," In: Cutler H, Cutler S eds. *Biologically Active Natural Products: Pharmaceuticals ACS Symposium Book. Boca Raton, LA,* 1999, CRC Press, 173-183.

Johnson, HA, Oberlies NH, Alali FQ, and McLaughlin JL, "Thwarting resistance: annonaceous acetogenins as new pesticidal and antitumor agents," *Biologically Active Natural Products: Pharmaceuticals ACS Symposium Book, Las Vegas, Nevada, eds. H. Cutler and S. Cutler, CRC Press, Boca Raton,* 1999, 173-183.

Landolt JL, Ahammadsahib KI, Hollingworth RM, Barr R, Crane FL, BuerckNL, McCabe GP, and McLaughlin JL, "Determination of structure-activity relationships of annonaceous acetogenins by inhibition of oxygen uptake in rat liver mitochondria," 1995, *Chemico-Biological Interactions,* 98 1-13.

Lewis MA, Arnason JL, Philogene BJR, Rupprecht JK, and McLaughlin JL, "Inhibition of respiration at site I by asimicin, an insecticidal acetogenin of the paw paw, Asimina triloba (Annonaceae)," *Pesticide Biochemistry and Physiology*, 1993, 45 (1):15-23.

Londershausen M, Leicht W, Lieb F, Moeschler H, Weiss H, "Molecular mode of action of annonins," *Pesticide Science*, 1991, 33 (4):427-438.

McLaughlin JL, Chang CJ, Smith DL, "Simple bench-top bioassays (brine shrimp and potato discs) for the discovery of plantantitumor compounds: review of recent progress," In: Kinghorn AD, Balandrin MF, eds. *Human Medicinal Agents from Plants, ACS Symposium Series 534. Washington, D.C.: American Chemical Society*, 1993, 112-137.

McLaughlin JL, Chang CJ, "Simple (bench-top) bioassays and the isolation of new chemically diverse antitumor and pesticidal agents from higher plants," In: Romeo JT, ed., *Recent Advances in Phytochemistry. New York: Kluwer Academic/Plenum Publishers*, 1999, 89-132.

McLaughlin JL, Rogers LL, Anderson JE, "The use of biological assays to evaluate botanicals," *Drug Information Journal*, 1998, 32 (2):513-524.

McLaughlin JL, Zeng L, Oberlies NH, Alfonso D, Johnson HA, Cummings BA, "Annonaceous acetogenins as new natural pesticides: recent progress," In: Hedin P, Hollingworth R, Mujamoto J, Mesler E, Thompson D, eds. *Phytochemical Pest Control Agents. Washington, D.C.: ACS Symposium*, 1997, 117-130.

McLaughlin JL, "Crown gall tumours in potato discs and brine shrimp lethality: two simple bioassays for higher plant screening and fractionation," In: Hostettmann K, ed. *Methods in Plant Biochemistry. London: Academic Press*, 1991, 1-31.

Miyoshi H, Ohshima M, Shimada H, Akazi T, Iwamura H, McLaughlin JL. "Essential structural factors of annonaceous acetogenins as potent inhibitors of mitochondrial complex 1," *Biochimica Biophysica Acta*, 1998, 1365 (3):443-452.

Morre DJ, de Cabo R, Farley C, Oberlies NH, McLaughlin JL, "Mode of action of bullatacin, a potent antitumor acetogenin: inhibition of NADH

oxidase activity of HELA and HL-60, but not liver, plasma membranes,"
Life Sciences, 1995 56 (5):343-348.

Morin MJ, "From oncogene to drug: development of small molecule
tyrosine kinase inhibitors and anti-tumor and anti-angiogenic agents," *Oncogene,* 2000, 19 6574-6583.

Moser TL, Stack MS, Asplin I, Enghild JJ, Hojrup P, Everitt L, Hub-
cnak S. Schnaper HW, and Pizzo SV "Angiostatin binds ATP synthase on
the surface of human endothelial cells," *Proceedings of the National Academy
of Sciences of the United States of America,* 1999, 96 2811-2816.

Oberlies NH, Alali FQ, McLaughlin JL. "Annonaceous acetogenins:
thwarting ATP dependent resistance,". In: Calls I, Ersoz T, Basaran AA, eds.
*New Trends and Methods in Natural Products Research, Proceedings of the 12"'
International Symposium on Plant Originated Crude Drugs, May 20-22, 1998.
Ankara, Turkey: The Scientific and Technical Research Council of Turkey,* 1999,
192-223.

Oberlies NH, Chang CJ, McLaughlin JL. "Structure-activity relationships of diverse annonaceous acetogenins against multidrug resistant human mammary adenocarcinoma (MCF7/adr) cells," *Journal of Medicinal
Chemistry,* 1997, 40 (13):2102-2106.

Oberlies NH, Croy VL, Harrison MH, McLaughlin JL. "The Annonaceous acetogenin bullatacin is cytotoxic against multidrug resistant human
mammary adenocarcinoma cells," *Cancer Letters,* 1997, 115 (1):173-179.

Oberlies NH, Jones JL, Corbett TH, Fotopoulos SS, McLaughlin JL.
"Tumor cell growth inhibition of annonaceous acetogenins in an in vitro
disk diffusion assay," *Cancer Letters,* 1995, 96 (1):55-62.

Oberlies, N.H., C.-J. Chang, and J.L. McLaughlin, "Structure-activity
relationships of diverse annonaceous acetogenins against multidrug resistant human mammary adenocarcinoma (MCF- 7/adr) cells," *Journal of Medicinal Chemistry,* 1997, 40 2102-2106.

Oberlies NH, Alali FQ, and McLaughlin JL, "Annonaceous acetogenins: thwarting ATP dependent resistance," in New Trends and Methods in Natural Products Research, eds. Calis I, Ersoz T, and Basaran AA, *Proceedings of the 12th International Symposium on Plant Originated Crude Drugs, May 20-22, 1998, The Scientific and Technical Research Council of Turkey. Ankara,* 1999, 192-223.

Oberlies NH, Jones JL, Corbett TH, Fotopoulos SS, McLaughlin JL, "Tumor cell growth inhibition of annonaceous acetogenins in an in vitro disk diffusion assay," *Cancer Letters,* 1995, 96 55- 62.

Oberlies, NH , Croy VL, Harrison MH, and McLaughlin JL, 'The Annonaceous acetogenin bullatacin is cytotoxic against multidrug resistant human mammary adenocarcinoma cells," *Cancer Letters,* 1997, 115 173-179.

Papa V, Pezzino V, Constantino A, Belfiore A, Giuffrida D, Frittitta L, Vannelli GB, Brand R, Goldfine ID, Vigneri R, "Elevated insulin receptor content in human breast cancer," *Journal of Clinical Investigation,* 1990, 86 (5): 1503-1510.

Ratnayake S, Gu ZM, Miesbauer LR, Smith DL, Wood KV, Evert DR, McLaughlin JL, "Parvifloracin and parviflorin: cytotoxic bis-tetrahydrofuran acetogenins with 35 carbons from Asimina parviflora (Annonaceae)," *Canadian Journal of Chemistry,* 1994, 72 (3):287-293.

Ratnayake S, Rupprecht JK, Potter WM, McLaughlin JL, "Evaluation of various parts of the paw paw tree, Asimina triloba (Annonaceae), as commercial sources of the pesticidal annonaceous acetogenins," *Journal of Economic Entomology,* 1992, 85 (6):2353-2356.

Rieser MJ, Hui YH, Rupprecht JK, Kozlowski JF, Wood KV, McLaughin JL, Hoye TR, Hanson PR, Zhuang ZP, "Determination of absolute configuration of stereogenic carbinol centers in annonaceous acetogenins by I H- and 1~~F- NMR analysis of Mosher ester derivatives," *Journal of the American Chemical Society,* 1992, 114 (26):10203-10213.

Rupprecht JK, Chang CJ, Cassady JM, McLaughlin JL, Mikolajczak KL, Weisleder D, "Asimicin, a new cytotoxic and pesticidal acetogenin from the paw paw, Asimina triloba (Annonaceae), *Heterocycles*, 1986, 24 (5):1197-1201.

Rupprecht JK, Hui YH, McLaughlin JL, "Annonaceous acetogenins: a review," *Journal of Natural Products*, 1990, 53 (2):237-278.

Rupprecht, JK, Chang CJ, Cassady JM, McLaughlin JL, Mikolajczak KL, and Weisleder D, "Asimicin, a new cytotoxic and pesticidal acetogenin from the paw paw, Asimina triloba (Annonaceae)," *Heterocycles*, 1986, 24 1197-1201.

Satake S, Kuzuya M, Miura H, Asai T, RamosMA, Muraguchi M, Ohmoto Y and Iguchi A, "Up-regulation of vascular endothelial growth factor in response to glucose deprivation," *Biology of the Cell*, 1998, 90 161 - 168.

Schuler F, Yano T, Di Bernardo S, Yagi T, Yankovskaya V, Singer TP, Casida JE, "NADHquinone oxidoreductase: PSST subunit couples electron transfer from iron-sulfur cluster N2 to quinone," *Proceedings of the National Academy of Sciences*, 1999, 96 (7):4149-53.

Shimada H, Grutzner JB, Kozlowski JF, McLaughlin JL, "Membrane conformations and their relation to cytotoxicity of asimicin and its analogues," *Biochemistry*, 1998, 37 (3):854-866.

Shimada H, Kozlowski JF, McLaughlin JL, "The localisations in liposomal membranes of the tetrahydrofuran ring moieties of the annonaceous acetogenins, annonacin and sylvaticin, as determined by 'H NMR spectroscopy," *Pharmacological Research*, 1998, 37 (5):357-384.

Shimada H, Grutzner JB, Kozlowski JF, and McLaughlin JL, "Membrane conformations and their relation to cytotoxicity of asimicin and its analogues," *Biochemistry*, 1998, 37 854-866.

Shimada H, Kozlowski JF, and McLaughlin JL, "The positions in liposomal membranes of the tetrahydrofuran ring moieties of the annonaceous acetogenins, annonacin and sylvaticin, as determined by NMR spectroscopy," *Pharmacological Research*, 1998, 37 357-384.

Woo MH, Cho KY, Zhang Y, Zeng L, Gu ZM, McLaughlin JL, "Asimilobin and cis- and trans-murisolinones, novel bioactive annonaceous acetogenins from the seeds of Asimina triloba," *Journal of Natural Products*, 1995, 58 (10):1533-1542.

Woo MH, Chung SO, Kim DH, "Asitrilobins C and D: two new cyto-toxic monotetrahydrofuran annonaceous acetogenins from Asimina triloba seeds," *Bioorganic and Medicinal Chemistry*, 2000 8 (1):285-290.

Woo MH, Kim DH, McLaughlin JL, "Asitrilobins A and B: cytotoxic mono-THF annonaceous acetogenins from the seeds of Asimina triloba,". *Phytochemistry*. 1999, 50 (6):1033-1040.

Woo MH, Zen L, Ye Q, Gu ZM, Zhao GX, McLaughlin JL, "16,19-cis-Murisolin and murisolin A, two novel bioactive mono-tetrahydrofuran an-nonaceous acetogenins from Asimina triloba seeds," *Bioorganic and Medici-nal Chemistry Letters*, 1995, 5 (11):1135-1140.

Woo MH, Zeng L, McLaughlin JL, "Asitribin and asimenins A and B, novel bioactive annonaceous acetogenins from the seeds of Asimina tri-loba," *Heterocycles*, 1995, 41 (8):1731-1742.

Ye Q, He K, Oberlies NH, Zeng L, Shi G, Evert D, McLaughlin JL, "Longimicins A-D: novel bioactive acetogenins from Asimina longifolia (Annonaceae) and structure-activity relationships of asimicin type annona-ceous acetogenins, *Journal of Medicinal Chemistry*,1996, 39 (9):1790-1796.

Ye Q, McLaughlin JL, Evert D, "bsolute stereochemistries of giganin and loganin, bioactive non-tetrahydrofuran ring annonaceous acetogenins from Asimina longifolia,"*Heterocycles*, 1996, 43 (8):1607-1512.

Zeng L, Ye Q, Oberlies NH, Shi G, Gu ZM, He K, McLaughlin JL, "Re-cent advances in annonaceous acetogenins," *Natural Product Reports*, 1996, 13 (4):275-306.

Zhao GX, Chao JF, Zeng L, McLaughlin JL, "(2,4-cis)-Asimicinone and (2,4-trcuzs)asimicinone: two novel ketolactone acetogenins fromAsimina triloba (Annonaceae)," *Natural Toxins*, 1996, 4 (3):128-134.

Zhao GX, Chao F, Zeng L, Rieser MJ, McLaughlinJL, "The absolute configuration of adjacent bis-THF acetogenins and asiminocin, a novel highly potent asimicin isomer from Asimina triloba," *Bioorganic and Medicinal Chemistry*, 1996, 4 (1):25-32.

Zhao GX, Gu ZM, Zen- L, Chao JF, Wood KV, Kozlowski JF, McLaughlin JL, "The absolute configuration of trilobacin and trilobin, a novel highly potent acetogenin from the stem bark of Asinzina triloba (Annonaceae)," *Tetrahedron*, 1995, 51 (26):7149-7160.

Zhao GX, Hui YH, Rupprecht JK, McLaughlin JL, Wood KV, "Additional bioactive compounds and trilobacin, a novel highly cytotoxic acetogenin, from the bark of Asimina triloba," *Journal of Natural Products*, 1992, 55 (3):347-356.

Zhao GX, Miesbauer LR, Smith DL, McLaughlin JL, "Asimin, asiminacin, and asiminecin: novel highly cytotoxic asimicin isomers from Asimina triloba," *Journal of Medicinal Chemistry*, 1994, 37 (13):1971-1976.

Zhao GX, Ng JH, Kozlowski JF, Smith DL, McLaughlin JL, "Bullatin and bullanin: two novel, highly cytotoxic acetogenins from Asimina triloba," *Heterocycles*, 1994, 38 (8):1897-1908.

Zhao GX, Rieser MJ, Hui YH, Miesbauer LR, Smith DL, McLaughlin JL, "Biologically active acetogenins from the stem bark of Asimina triloba," *Phytochemistry*, 1993, 33 (5):10651073.

Zhao GX, Hui YH, Rupprecht JK, McLaughlin JL, and Wood KV, "Additional bioactive compounds and trilobacin, a novel highly cytotoxic acetogenin, from the bark of Asimina triloba," *Journal of Natural Products*, 1992, 55 347-356.

Zhao, GX, Gu ZM, Zeng L, Chao JF, Wood KV, Kozlowski JF, and McLaughlin JL, "The absolute configuration of trilobacin and trilobin, a novel highly potent acetogenin from the stem bark of Asimina triloba (Annonaceae)," *Tetrahedron*, 1995, 51 7149-7160.

Internet

Sites with General Information about Paw Paw and Cancer.

Asterisks (*) indicate sites of special interest:

http://alternativecancer.us

http://cancer-cures-plus.com/?page_id=504 (*)
(very good - about MDR cells and paw paw)

http://pawpawresearch.com

http://thetruthaboutcancer.com/

http://ww3.curecancercells.com/

http://www.cancer.gov/

http://www.canceractive.com/ (UK site)

http://www.cancertutor.com/graviola/ (*)

http://www.collective-evolution.com/category/health/

http://www.livescience.com/health/

http://www.mnwelldir.org/docs/cancer1/pawpaw.htm

http://www.naturopathic.org/

http://www.navigatelungcancer.bmsinformation.com/emerging-research

http://www.nih.gov/news/health/archives/index.htm
(searchable site, all health issues)

http://www.pawpaws.net/

http://www.secondopinionnewsletter.com

http://www.self-helpcancer.org/optionsaz.htm (*)

http://www.smashcancer.com/tag/paw-paw/

http://www.thedoctorwithin.com/cancer/to-the-cancer-patient/

http://www.treelite.com/downloads/PawPaw.pdf (*)

https://www.youtube.com/watch?v=NAMYAoiCSsI
   (Video. Controversial use of sodium bicarbonate to
   cure cancer)

Scientific Articles about Paw Paw - Free online versions

http://www.pawpawresearch.com/pawpaw-trials1.pdf

http://www.ncbi.nlm.nih.gov/pmc/articles/PMC3672862/

http://www.rain-tree.com/plantdrugs.htm#.VOoOlS69gk5

http://www.pawpaw.kysu.edu/PDF/McLaughlin2008.pdf

http://www.pawpaws.net/Pawpaw_Scientific_Paper.htm

https://www.burtongoldberg.com/home/burtongoldberg/contribution-of-chemotherapy-to-five-year-survival-rate-morgan.pdf

Acknowledgements

There are so many people who helped and supported me in this effort that it's hard to know where to begin in expressing my gratitude. Needless to say, my wife Josée's fortitude, patience, and endurance was an inspiration to me. I simply could not have written this book without her. An author herself, Josée's advice was, as usual, treasured. I especially want to thank my friend Al Parinello, who helped me in so many ways that I wouldn't attempt to enumerate them. His counsel and devotion to the project have been invaluable. Don Hauptman's sharing of his expertise and resources are also greatly appreciated.

Then there were the many, many donors to our crowdfunding campaign whose belief in the books' success translated into real financial help in the publicity and promotion of the book.

And lastly, a "thank you" to all the participants in the many studies of paw paw, and the medical professionals who conducted those studies and contributed to the vast body of knowledge from which I drew the information that appears within these covers.

About the Author

John Clifton[56] became an author when he co-wrote a book with his wife Josée Clerens, *Sparky Fights Back: A Little Dog's Big Battle Against Cancer*.[57] This best-seller chronicled the miraculous survival of their lymphoma-stricken pet. In 2007 he authored *Stop the Shots! Are Vaccinations Killing Our Pets?* That highly researched work, which investigated the pros and cons of animal vaccines, became the most popular book on the topic, and remains so to this day. When his wife contracted Stage IV lung cancer in 2012, John began intensive research on alternative cancer treatments. The result of this wealth of research and Josée's exceptional outcome led him to write the present volume.

John has had a long and varied career as an artist, writer, composer, lyricist, musician, teacher, and investigative journalist. Trained as a graphic artist (BFA Carnegie Melon 1957), John worked in advertising in his post-college years, only to switch to music in 1962, and continued to write and compose for the theater for most of his life. Having written dozens of musicals, his work has been presented on Broadway, off-Broadway, television, and recordings. Later in life he taught in professional and private schools.

Index

Also from **Foley Square Books** . . .

Buying Louisiana
An Eyewitness's Account of the Louisiana Purchase
by Josée Clerens
BuyingLouisiana.com

Stop the Shots!
Are Vaccinations Killing Our Pets?
By John Clifton
StopTheShots.com

Sparky Fights Back
A Little Dog's Big Battle Against Cancer
by Josée Clerens and John Clifton
SparkyFightsBack.com

The Forbidden Political Dictionary
Complete and Unapproved
by John Clifton
ForbiddenDictionary.com

Man with a Load of Mischief
The Complete Script of the Musical
by Ben Tarver and John Clifton
MischiefTheMusical.com

Man with a Load of Mischief
The Complete Piano/Vocal Score
by John Clifton and Ben Tarver
MischiefTheMusical.com

To order additional copies of this book, simply fill in this
form and mail with payment.
(or order at YourFourthChoice.com)

Please send me ____copies of
*Your Fourth Choice: Killing Cancer Cells with Paw Paw
—that Little-Known Treatment that Grows on Trees*

Normally ships via USPS Mail.
<u>Note</u>: US and Canadian orders only. Other countries please pur-
chase online at <u>*www.YourFourthChoice.com*</u>

PLEASE PRINT CLEARLY:

How many copies?	**Cost** ($21.95 + $2.00 S/H **per copy**)	Total Enclosed (Check or Money Order Only)
	x $23.95	

Full Name	
Address 1	
Address 2	
City	State
Zip Code	
Email	
Telephone (day): [ ] [ ]	
Area Number	

Send to:
Foley Square Books
175 West 87th Street, Room 27E
New York, NY 10024